SEVERE BURNS

A Family Guide to Medical and Emotional Recovery

Andrew M. Munster, M.D.
and the Staff of the
Baltimore Regional Burn Center

The care of severe burn victims—over 100,000 people are hospitalized each year—has improved dramatically over the past fifty years. But a serious burn remains a painful, frightening, and traumatic experience. The psychological stress of injury may be increased by the formidable array of medical equipment used in the early stages of care and by the number of doctors, nurses, and specialists that burn patients and their families encounter. Once out of intensive care, the burn survivor often faces a long and difficult recovery.

This book is meant to relieve some of the confusion and anxiety that comes with any serious burn injury. Written by the staff of the Baltimore Regional Burn Center, it includes comprehensive medical information from leading experts—and first-person accounts of the experiences of burn survivors. The book describes the different types of burns, the various stages of treatment and recovery, the roles of all the people on the "burn team," the physical and emotional challenges of rehabilitation, and the resources available to patients and families. It also explains how to prevent injuries in the future and how to administer first aid to someone who has been burned.

SEVERE BURNS

SEVERE BURNS

A Family Guide to Medical and Emotional Recovery

Andrew M. Munster, M.D.
and the Staff of the
Baltimore Regional Burn Center

The Johns Hopkins University Press
Baltimore and London

Note to the Reader

This book is not meant to substitute for medical care of people with burn injuries. Instead, treatment must be developed by medical professionals, with the participation of the patient and the patient's family.

In this book, brand names are used when no appropriate generic term is available. Use of such names does not constitute a recommendation for the use of a particular product or brand of product.

Illustrations by Timothy H. Phelps, M.S., FAMI

Printed in the United States of America on acid-free paper

The Johns Hopkins University Press
2715 North Charles Street
Baltimore, Maryland 21218-4319
The Johns Hopkins Press Ltd., London

Library of Congress Cataloging-in-Publication Data

Munster, Andrew M., 1935–
Severe burns ; a family guide to medical and emotional recovery / Andrew M. Munster and the staff of the Baltimore Regional Burn Center.
p. cm.
Includes index.
ISBN 0-8018-4653-6 (acid-free paper)
1. Burns and scalds—Patients—Rehabilitation. 2. Burns and scalds—Treatment. I. Baltimore Regional Burn Center. II. Title.
RD96.4.M867 1993
617.1'103—dc20 93-870

A catalog record for this book is available from the British Library.

Contents

Figures

Tables

Contributors

Earl W. Brooks
Fire Marshall
Francis Scott Key Medical Center

Mary E. Clark, RN
Nursing Educator IV
Baltimore Regional Burn Center

LaWanda Conaway
Therapeutic Cosmetician
Baltimore Regional Burn Center

Ceal Curry, B.S., CCLS
Child Life Therapist
Francis Scott Key Medical Center

Diane Blake Doyle, OTR/L
Baltimore Regional Burn Center

James A. Fauerbach, Ph.D.
Chief Psychologist
Baltimore Regional Burn Center and the Center for Burn Reconstruction
and Instructor in Division of Medical Psychology
The Johns Hopkins Medical School

Cynthia R. Fisher, EMT-A
Nursing Unit Secretary

Mary E. Frank, RN
Baltimore Regional Burn Center

Linda French, PT
Baltimore Regional Burn Center and Mid-Atlantic Burn Camp Director

Gail Horowitz, M.S.W.

E. Tonas Kalil, PT
Baltimore Regional Burn Center

Andrew M. Munster, M.D.
Director
Baltimore Regional Burn Center
and Professor of Surgery and Plastic Surgery
The Johns Hopkins Medical School

Dianna Murray, RN
Baltimore Regional Burn Center

Lana Parsons, M.S., ANP-C
Burn Trauma Coordinator
Baltimore Regional Burn Center

Margaret A. Schmitt, M.S., PT
Burn Rehabilitation Manager
Baltimore Regional Burn Center

Melissa Smith-Meek, B.S.
Clinical Research Coordinator
Baltimore Regional Burn Center

Robert J. Spence, M.D.
Codirector
Baltimore Regional Burn Center
Chief
Division of Plastic and Reconstructive Surgery
Director
Center for Burn Reconstruction
and Assistant Professor of Plastic Surgery
The Johns Hopkins Medical School

Gerrie Stancik, M.S.W., LCSW
Clinical Social Worker
Baltimore Regional Burn Center

Beth Ann Sutcliffe-Basham, OTR/L
Baltimore Regional Burn Center

Linda Coll Ware, OTR/L
Baltimore Regional Burn Center

Ilene P. Wiggins, RN
Baltimore Regional Burn Center

Lesley Wong, M.D.
Assistant Director
Baltimore Regional Burn Center
and Assistant Professor of Plastic Surgery
The Johns Hopkins Medical School

BURN SURVIVORS

Bob Campbell

Bryan Haines

Annie Kuebler

Caroline C. Rouen

Preface

This book was written especially for you. You may be a burn survivor, though you may also be thinking of yourself as a burn patient. Or you may be a burn survivor's wife, husband, mother, father, sister, brother, daughter, son, fiancé, or friend. You have a special interest in burns, because you or someone close to you has been injured.

Reading this book will help sort out some of the confusion in what's going on around you, and perhaps it will relieve some of your anxiety and fears as well. Not only will it help explain what's happening now, it will also help you know what's likely to happen over the long run. Think of this book as a survivor's handbook, if you will, and let it take you step by step through the recovery process.

This book will explain everything that takes place during recovery, starting at the time the burn injury occurs. It will dispel some of the mystery about what's going on behind the closed doors of the emergency room. It will describe the different kinds of burn injury and how wounds are treated in the first weeks after injury (Chapter 1). It will explain the roles of all the people who make up the burn team as well as their equipment (Chapter 3). It will guide you through the absolute pure effort of rehabilitation (Chapter 4), the trips to surgery (Chapter 6), and the hours of waiting. It will let you know what resources are available to help you and your family heal (Chapter 7 and Appendixes B and C). It will tell you how to prevent burn injuries in the future (Chapter 8) and how to administer first aid to someone who has been burned (Appendix A).

But this book doesn't focus only on the physical aspects of recovery. We know that a major burn injury is also a devastating event emotionally. Bewilderment, fear, anger, guilt, and concerns about the future dominate at this time. The injury may have involved significant property loss, with all the financial implications that accompany the loss. Chapter 2 tells family and friends of the burn patient how they can help in the recovery of the burn patient as well as how they themselves can cope with the changes the injury of a loved one will bring to their lives. Chapter 5 will help the burn survivor deal with the psychological and social issues he or she will encounter in the hospital, at home, and out in the world.

Being a burn survivor means so much more than simply being alive. Being a burn survivor also means being a take-charge-of-your-life person whose strength of spirit is inspirational to others. Burn survivors have to learn to accept that life as they knew it before the injury is lost. With this acceptance comes profound grief, of course, but many burn survivors grow to a level of personal awareness and acceptance of self that most people never experience.

One burn survivor says that, for her, being burned is like having a bad dream, but you never wake up. In the dream you're looking down at yourself only to see that your body is all scarred, but you feel the same inside. What an awful dream. You can't wait to wake up. For burn survivors this dream never stops; it is their reality.

In this book you will find the personal stories of four people involved in burn injury. *These stories are the highlight of our book. Whatever else you may be interested in that is contained in this volume, these stories are must reading. The stories were brought together by LaWanda Conaway, herself a burn survivor and now a Burn Center staff member. We are most grateful to her and her colleagues for allowing us to share their experiences. The words are their own; nothing has been changed.*

Reading these stories may take you through a whirlwind of emotions, and parts of the stories may make you uncomfortable, but we ask you, please, to read each story in its entirety. All of the stories have an ending that can inspire you.

Introduction

The Who, Where, and How of Burn Injury

Fire is the fourth greatest cause of accidental death in the United States. It is surpassed only by motor vehicle accidents, falls, and drowning as a cause of unintentional injury death. Each year, an estimated 20,000 adults and children die, and an additional 75,000 to 100,000 are hospitalized, from fire-related injuries. Each year more than a million burn injuries require medical care or restriction of activity. Burn injuries occur in house fires, auto accidents, and work-related accidents, as well as in recreational accidents involving campfires, outdoor grills, boats, aircraft, and motorcycles. In short, anything that involves heat, chemicals, or fires can cause a burn injury.

The most common cause of burn injury is flame, and the most common place of injury is the home (Figures I.1 and I.2). In fact, house fires cause three-fourths of all fire injuries. Very young children and older people are injured in house fires more frequently and more seriously than other people, perhaps because both the very young and the very elderly have difficulty escaping. Inhalation injury to the respiratory tract is also common and more serious in these fires, which occur in a closed space.

Males are more likely than females to be injured in a fire (males account for 74 percent of burn injuries). This may be because boys play with matches more often than girls do, and because more men than women have jobs with a high risk of burn injury from contact with steam, chemicals, electricity, fire, and explosive materials. After the home, the workplace is the second most common place for burn injury to occur. Because of this, adults experience more burn injuries (63 percent) than children (37 percent).

Scalds are the second leading cause of burn injury. Children and the elderly are more likely to receive scald burns than people in the

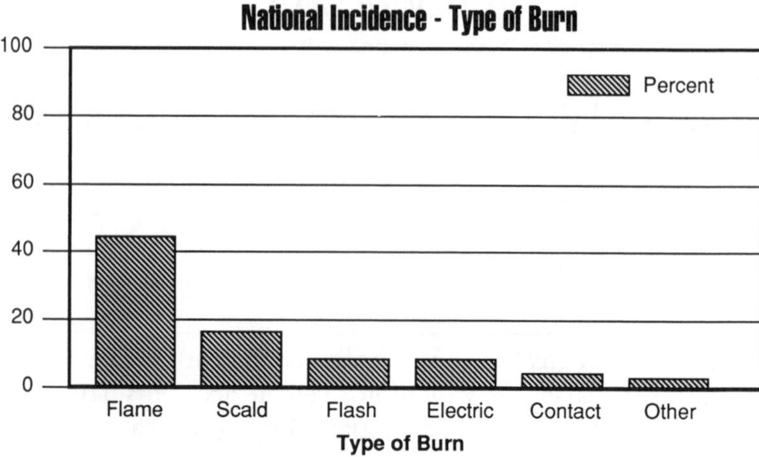

Figure I.1. National Incidence: Type of Burn-causing Injury

other age groups, and contact with hot liquids is the most common cause of hospitalized burns among children and the elderly. A hot pot or cup of hot coffee might get pulled over accidentally, or the person may slip in the tub and land in water that is too hot. By lowering the temperature in the hot-water system in the home and in public buildings, the potential for scalds is reduced. If the hot-water heater setting is turned up to 159°F, for example, it takes one second—the time required to snap your fingers—for a full-thickness (through all the layers of the skin) burn to occur. At a setting of 120°F it would take *three minutes* for this to happen, perhaps just enough time to avoid injury. To put this into perspective, consider that a slow "crock pot"–type cooker cooks on low at 140°F and on high at 180°F. It's easy to see that 120°F is hot enough for household water. Another source of scald injury is the radiator in the family car. Cars overheat in winter as well as in summer, and people sometimes make the mistake of taking the safety cap off while the steam is still hissing out around it.

Another type of injury which is often not thought of as a burn injury (though it certainly is) is the electrical injury. Electrical injury accounts for about 3 percent of all burns. An electrical injury can result from direct contact, an arc, or a flame. It can occur at home, at work, or in the community. It can be anything from a simple "tingle" in your fingertips that makes you take notice, to a

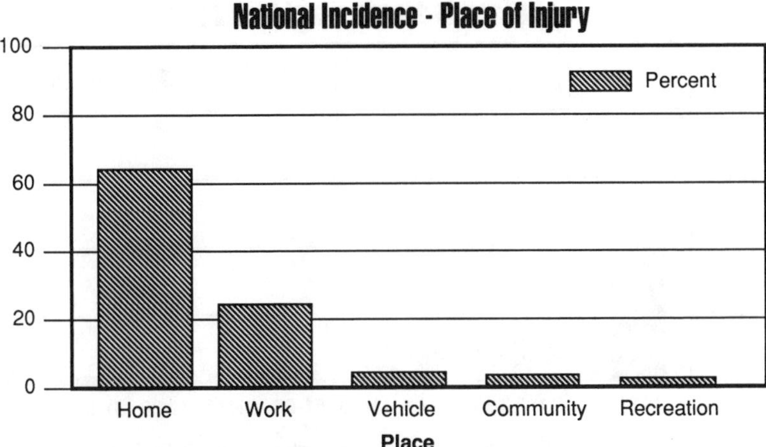

Figure I.2. National Incidence: Place of Injury

major life-threatening event. Contact with electricity can damage many body systems, including blood vessels, tendons, nerves, muscles, bone, soft tissues, the heart, the eyes, the kidneys, and the skin. It is very difficult to tell at first just how much damage has been done, because electrical injuries are often progressive. That is, it takes some time for the damage to complete its course. This explains why the hospital staff will tell a person who has just been injured by coming into contact with electricity that it will be some time before the full extent of the injury can be determined. The staff knows that the waiting and not knowing is hard for the patient and the family, but they also know that it can take three weeks or so for the extent of injuries to become clear.

A small percentage of patients treated in burn centers are patients with chemical injuries. Chemical injuries usually fall into two types: occupational and those occurring in the home. Chemical injuries at home are usually minor, whereas occupational injury from chemicals may be more severe. They frequently occur in steel mills, foundries, oil refineries, and chemical plants. Chemical injuries are limited to the area of contact, unless the chemical has been absorbed into the person's system. The strength of the chemical and the duration of contact determine the extent of injury from chemical exposure.

Smoke inhalation or inhalation injury is not a burn per se, but it

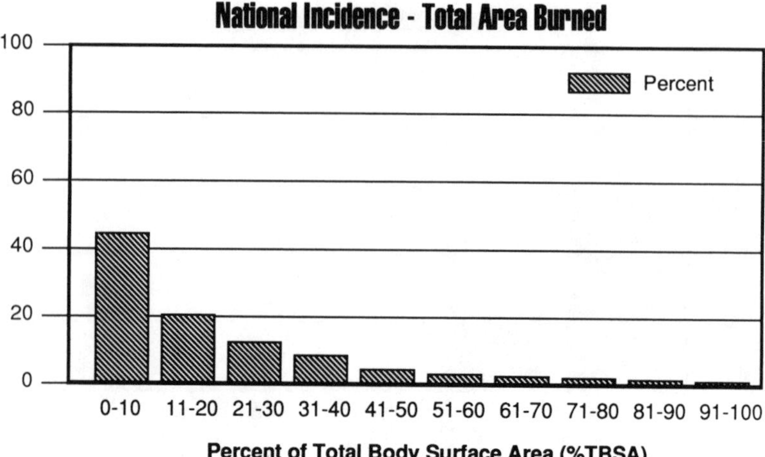

Figure I.3. National Incidence: Total Area Burned

is a very serious complication of many burn injuries. About 5 percent of all burn injuries involve smoke inhalation. Smoke inhalation usually occurs during a fire contained in a closed space, where smoke and heat are concentrated. It would be more likely to occur in a house fire when someone is inside (a closed space) than outside while someone is burning leaves, for example. It can also occur during a chemical fire, when toxic fumes are inhaled and the respiratory tract is damaged. The inhalation injury may be mild or severe. A very mild injury might just require taking oxygen by a mask for a few days, whereas a severe injury might require having a breathing tube inserted into the trachea.

About half of all burn injuries involve 10 percent or less of the body surface (Figure I.3). Another third of the injuries involve from 11 to 30 percent of the body surface. These are encouraging figures, because these figures, along with tremendous improvements in medical care, mean that most people with burn injuries will survive. This means that fire prevention education is working, that improved firefighting techniques are working, and that people with serious burns are surviving more often than in the past.

Other factors affecting survival include the victim's underlying health, vigor, and attitude. We know of a man who was a prisoner of war in Burma during World War II. Several thousand prisoners starved, and several thousand prisoners developed all kinds of diseases. The difference between those who made it and those who didn't, he said, was often the *will.* People on the burn team recognize that the will to survive affects the outcome for a burn survivor, too. It's exactly the same thing.

Part I

The Early Course of Burn Treatment

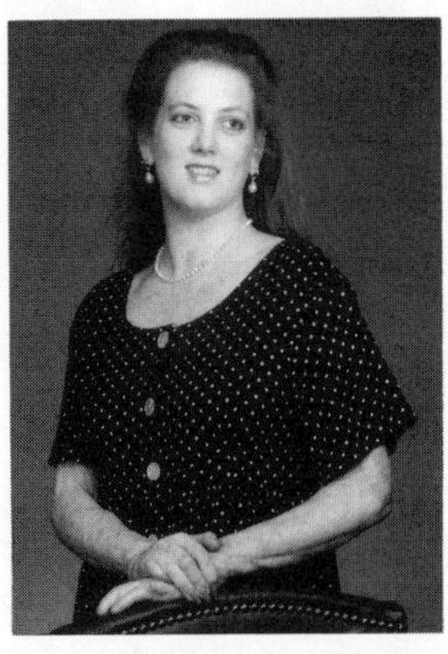

After August 20, 1987, my life would never be the same again. A newspaper article published a year after I was burned described the events of that day as follows:

> Caroline C. Rouen sat in the third floor window as the heat charred her body and flames rampaged through the Harrisburg townhouse, shattering windows and mangling doors. She realized only one thing could save her life: Jump.
>
> She landed on her feet, on concrete. The impact broke every bone in her feet and fractured a bone in her back. The burns were worse . . . they almost killed her.

This particular newspaper article related all of my successes and achievements over the year since the fire. They were accomplishments and achievements that I never thought would happen. They were dreams come true. Getting there wasn't easy. It was hell.

The fire on August 20, 1987, left me with third-degree burns over 65 percent of my body. Both of my arms and hands were burned. I lost the fingertips and most of my pinky on my left hand. My entire back was burned and parts of my legs. Every week I went to the operating room to have another part of my body repaired. The good skin I had left on my legs was being used to cover the areas that had been burned. I began to feel like a patchwork quilt.

At the time of my injury I was headed into my junior year of college. I was ready to dive back into the books, live in my first real apartment, and attend all the college football games, parties, and events that most college students do. My burn injury wasn't in the plan for me. The day classes started I was fighting for my life in the Baltimore Regional Burn Center.

Of the 18 weeks I spent in the Burn Unit, there is very little I remember. I do remember that all at once there were people constantly at my side, poking, prodding, drawing blood, touching me and moving me in ways I never wanted to be touched or moved. I couldn't voice any of my thoughts, but I just seemed too exhausted to care. Day in and day out it was pain and more pain. I wanted to take a shower so much—but what I wanted more than that was just not to move.

I was bedridden due to my broken back for at least three months. I lay in two positions. On my face or on my back. The position depended on what part of my body had been worked on in the operating room that week. I was log rolled for dressing changes. This was also when my lungs got the best workout, because I was a screamer. I honestly believe that my hospital "family" loved me and hated me. All anyone had to do was walk into my room and my lungs ripped. I was lucky not to have had any smoke inhalation. It was to my advantage—and to the burn staff's advantage. In retrospect, I believe it was more fear than pain that caused me to scream and the nurses to wear cotton in their ears. The pain was inevitable, but the fear made it worse.

I believe my biggest fears stemmed from having absolutely no control over what was happening to me. I had no idea what being burned meant. I did not understand the procedures that were being performed on me, and I was too afraid to ask where, specifically, I was burned. I had no say when it came to my care. I just had to comply with the doctors and nurses and deal with things as they arose. I was forced into trusting people I had never met—with my life. Unfortunately, I was not very compliant. I fought and screamed every chance I had. I felt that all these people taking care of me were more concerned with my physical recovery than with what was going on in my mind. I literally felt trapped; there was no way out. All I could do was wait. And heal.

The burn nurses are those very special people whom a burn patient tends to hate on a daily basis. It's hard to understand that the people doing all those painful procedures aren't there to cause pain but to help you heal. Burn nurses also have an unusual way of making you feel safe in what I often viewed as hell on earth. Throughout nightmares, loneliness, fear, and a never-ending stream of questions a nurse is there . . . 24 hours a day.

As a burn survivor, visiting hours are the one thing there is to look forward to every day, and I did. At least one member of my family made the one and a half hour trip to visit me on a daily basis. My mother and father often brought tea. My sister and her fiancé brought McDonald's or Pizza Hut, and my brother brought himself from New Jersey almost every weekend. It really wasn't food or drink that mattered but company. Someone to be there when I woke up from surgery or from sleep. Someone to calm me when I was afraid. Someone who loved me. Sometimes just having someone there made all the difference in the world. Just so I wasn't alone.

When my family wasn't by my side at the hospital, I knew they were thinking of me and praying for me at all times. They kept me informed of everything that was going on at home or in the neighborhood. They told me daily which friends or extended family had called to check on my progress. Although many of my college acquaintances went on with their lives, I had one special friend who called me weekly and sent me many cards. His family also stayed well informed of my progress. With people like that on my side, the encumbrance of the burns became lighter.

The daily process of healing was not pleasant. It seemed just when I got used to one procedure, they changed it. Just when I started to trust the new residents, they left. Just when one part of me healed, another needed healing. It seemed a never-ending process, and I continuously wondered if I'd ever be "normal" again. Who was going to love me? And, would I be alone for the rest of my life?

As far as answering those questions, I think I just stopped asking. I began to believe that they were not even relevant because, in time, I began to believe what people had been telling me all along. I was still the same person inside. Looking in a mirror, that was difficult to accept. I felt everything I was, was gone. The facts were I became as "normal" as I wanted to be and, in time, I felt like my old self again with many additional improvements. The people who loved me before I got burned loved me after. Those who left, although it was difficult, I came to believe that they didn't appreciate me as much as I thought they had. And as for being alone, I never was.

When I left the Burn Unit two days before Christmas, a whole new well of fears built up inside. I realized how very well the staff had taken care of me. I was fearful of leaving because I wasn't sure if I would receive such care and understanding anywhere else. Even at home. The reality for that situation was that the Burn Staff worked with my family to prepare them for how to take care of me at home. They did a fantastic job.

When I left the Burn Unit, I had many operations ahead of me, and a long way to go before I was going to consider myself physically recovered. I typically would not wear any clothing that would reveal my burned arms, legs, or back, and the thought of a bathing suit was not even conceivable. I spent a lot of time feeling sorry for myself, which never got me anywhere. What did get me somewhere was resuming my life where I left off wherever possible. I kept up with operations and therapy while I went back to school, and I graduated only one year late. I then went on to graduate school.

After leaving the Burn Unit, it became apparent that there weren't too many people in my life who really understood what was going on in my mind. I had outstanding support from family and many friends, but there were still questions that only other burn survivors could answer. It didn't take too long before I became aware of the burn survivor's support group at the Burn Unit. In that room, we could share our experiences, strengths, hopes, fears, and concerns and be understood like no one else could understand us. Sharing my experiences and feelings with other survivors helped me realize I wasn't alone. There are many survivors out there a lot like me. For a long time I thought I was the only female, 20-year-old burn survivor in the world.

If there's one thing I would tell a person just entering the new way of life, I believe it would be to never give up on yourself. Daily, a burn survivor may want to give up, but by hanging on to dreams and believing in yourself to make it, making it through becomes reality. I did it and, one day at a time, you can, too.

Caroline C. Rouen

Chapter 1

Critical Burn Care

Because each patient is an individual, there aren't any general rules that can be applied to every patient or to every burn injury. But the course of treatment—and healing—following a major burn injury can be *described* in a general way, and that is the approach we take in this chapter. Our purpose here is to outline what can be expected immediately after a burn injury.

You may want to consider this chapter an extension of what the primary care physician may tell a family during their first meeting. It provides answers to the questions most frequently asked by the family in this initial meeting.

The First Step: Assessing Life-threatening Conditions

Most people, when first thinking about a burn, worry about scarring and appearance; the possibility of death seems remote. Yet survival is clearly the first priority: despite advances in treatment and care, people do die from burn injury and its complications. That's why members of the medical team will evaluate the patient's vital signs before they do anything else.

The medical team's first concern is not the burn wound itself but the patient's life-sustaining systems of respiration and blood circulation. The physicians' initial evaluations will focus on determining whether the patient has shock or respiratory insufficiency, either of which may be immediately life-threatening.

Shock is defined as a decreased rate of circulation to vital organs; if an inadequate amount of blood is circulating to these organs, they are being deprived of the oxygen they need to function.

The severity of shock generally correlates with the amount of the body that has been burned, expressed as a percentage of the entire body surface area. If this percentage is significant, if there are other medical problems, or if smoke inhalation is suspected, the patient will probably be monitored in an intensive care unit. He or she will be connected to a heart monitor and may have a catheter placed directly into an artery or into the heart so pressure can be continually monitored.

Shock is detected by measuring the patient's blood pressure, pulse, and urine output. Treatment consists primarily of giving fluids by vein (intravenously). The amount of fluid needed is calculated for each individual and is based on the patient's weight and the amount of body area that has been burned. If the shock is severe, or if there are associated medical problems, especially cardiac problems, it may be necessary to administer medications by vein.

Respiratory insufficiency is defined as the inability of the lungs to supply enough oxygen to the body. This condition is more likely if the patient has smoke inhalation. Smoke inhalation may be suspected if the burn occurred in a closed space, if the patient has facial burns, or if soot is present in the nose or throat. Respiratory insufficiency can have a *delayed onset,* meaning it occurs some time after the initial injury, or it may worsen during the patient's hospital stay.

Poisonous gases from burning materials, especially plastics, cause lung injury from smoke inhalation. If carbon monoxide is present in the smoke, the patient will not be alert and may go into a coma. In addition to damaging the lungs and impairing the lungs' ability to provide sufficient oxygen to the bloodstream, the toxins from burning materials and the heat of inhaled smoke can also burn and cause swelling of the air passages themselves. This causes the air passages to narrow, and they may partially or completely close off. To avoid asphyxiation, immediate treatment is necessary.

To determine the presence and severity of smoke inhalation, physicians may run a number of tests, including chest x-rays, measuring the amount of oxygen in the blood, calculating the level of breathing function (*spirometry*), and looking into the nasal and lung air passages with a lighted flexible scope (*bronchoscopy* or *nasopharyngoscopy*). The primary treatment for smoke inhalation is administration of supplemental oxygen, initially given by face mask. If this is not adequate to supply sufficient levels of oxygen, or if there is swelling of the air passages, the patient may need to be placed on a ventilator through a tube in the mouth or nose entering the windpipe. If the respiratory insufficiency is severe or prolonged, a *tracheostomy* may be performed, in which a tube is surgically placed directly into the windpipe through the neck (see Chapter 3).

What factors affect survival?

The first determinant of survival is *burn size,* measured as a percentage of the total body surface involved. Burns involving more than 20 percent of the body surface (less in small babies) or any deep (third-degree) burns over 10 percent of the body surface are classified as critical by the American Burn Association. Certain chemical and high-voltage electrical burns are also classified as critical. Persons with burns classified as critical are best cared for in a burn unit (see Chapter 3). In addition, even small burns of the hands, face, feet, and genitalia are best taken care of in a burn unit, not because of their severity but because burns in these areas may impair function and appearance.

As the burn size increases, the chances of survival diminish. With burns over 90 percent of the body, even though spectacular survivals are now frequently recorded, the chances of survival are slight.

The *third-degree component,* or how much of the *total* burn is third-degree burn, also affects survival. A 50 percent all third-degree burn, or even a mixed-degree burn, is much more serious than a 50 percent all second-degree burn.

Age is another determinant of survival. In terms of the body's response to injury in general and burns in particular, aging begins at 35. By age 50, the ability to heal and fight infection is quite diminished. A 30 percent burn in a person who is 80 years old is as life-threatening as an 80 percent burn in a 20-year-old.

The person's *general physical condition* affects the outcome of burn injury, as it affects the outcome of so many injuries and illnesses. The strength of the person's *will to live* is also frequently a factor in survival.

Finally, *smoke inhalation* and *shock* determine a person's immediate chances for survival after a burn injury.

Generally the younger and more fit the patient is, and the smaller the burn is, the better the chances for survival—if smoke inhalation is not severe. With advancing age, illness, and smoke inhalation, chances for survival diminish progressively. The treating physicians may or may not feel comfortable predicting the outcome, as each patient is unique and each patient's recovery is unpredictable.

Step Two: Burn Assessment

Once vital signs and functions are stabilized, the medical team turns its attention to assessing the burn injury itself. Burns are judged by the *size of the burn* in relation to the whole body and by the *depth of the burn* (determined by how much of the thickness of the skin is involved). The size of the burn is described as a percentage of the total body surface area. The palm of your hand, for example, is equal to about 1 percent of your body's surface area.

The body can be divided into areas equaling multiples of 9 percent of the total body surface area by the "Rule of Nines." The head and arms are each equal to 9 percent of the body surface. The chest and back are each 18 percent (2×9 percent). Each leg is 18 percent (2×9 percent). This totals eleven nines, or 99 percent. The head of infants and small children is a relatively larger proportion of the total body surface area and the limbs relatively smaller than in adults (Figure 1.1).

How *deep* is the burn? Burn depth is measured in terms of "degrees" (Figure 1.2). To understand this measuring system, it is helpful to understand something about the structure of normal skin (see Figure 6.4). The outermost layer is the *epidermis*, which is composed of living keratinocytes and melanocytes, the pigment cells that impart color to the skin. As old epidermal cells die off, new cells replace them. Under the epidermis is the thicker layer of skin, called the *dermis*, which is largely made of the protein collagen. Blood vessels, nerves, oil glands, hair follicles, and sweat glands are located in this layer. The cells that regenerate skin line the hair follicles and sweat glands. Thus, these "accessory structures" are necessary for the skin to be able to "heal itself."

The purpose of skin is to limit the loss of water, electrolytes, and proteins from the body and to act as a barrier to bacterial invasion.

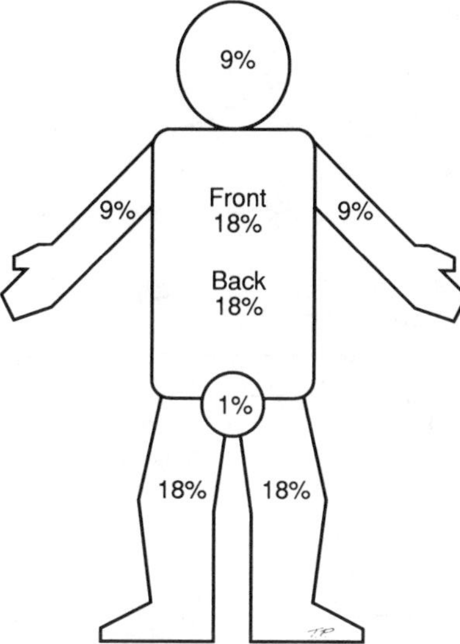

Figure 1.1. The "Rule of Nines" allows health care professionals to make a rapid estimation of the percentage of total body surface area that has been injured.

When skin is damaged in a burn, sensation may be altered along with sweating function and possibly hair growth. Damaged skin also results in loss of fluid and entrance of bacteria into deeper layers of skin and even into the body.

A first-degree burn is superficial, involving injury only to the outermost layer of skin—the epidermis—and is like a sunburn. The skin becomes red, warm, swollen, and painful. The skin may even peel, but the damage to the skin heals within a few days, by a process called *epithelialization* (see Chapter 6). A first-degree burn is sometimes called an *epidermal burn.*

Second-degree burns are caused by brief contact with fire and by scalds from liquids that are mostly water, such as tea and coffee. A second-degree burn involves a portion of the dermis as well as the epidermis—this is called a partial-thickness burn. It can range from superficial to deep partial thickness, depending on how many of the epidermal accessory structures are left in the remaining dermis. The skin is blistered, moist, discolored, and painful.

Spontaneous healing is possible, usually within four to six weeks. Occasionally the medical team will recommend skin graft-

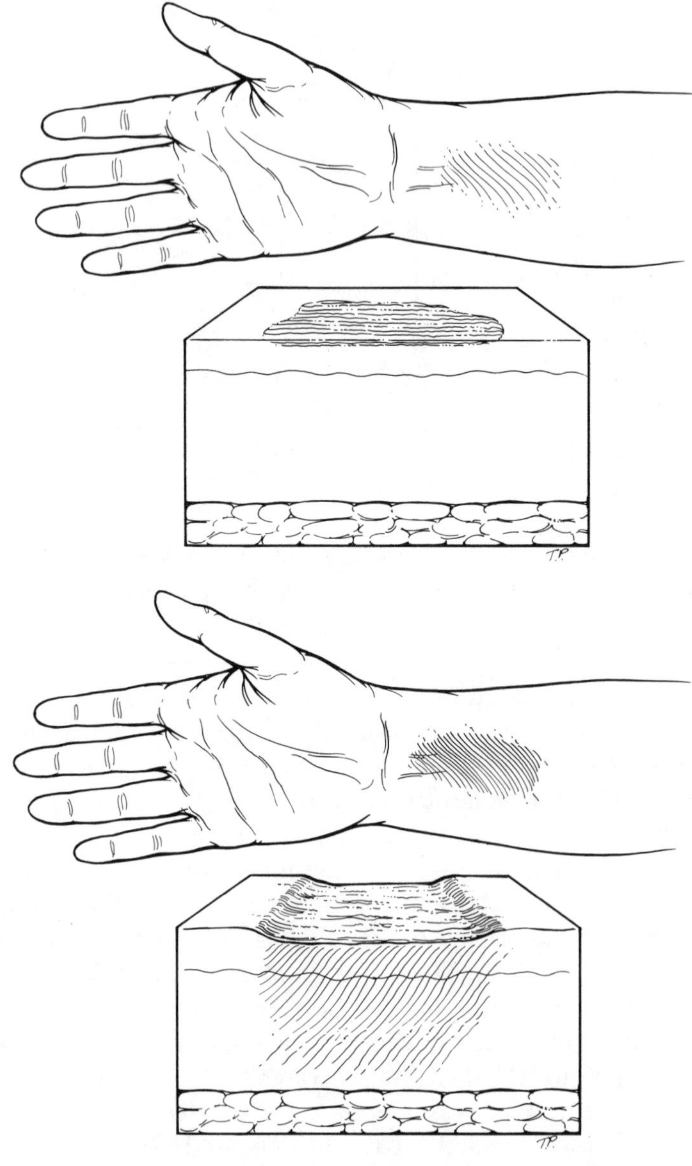

Figure 1.2. A first-degree, or epidermal, burn (*top left*); a superficial second-degree burn, also called a superficial partial-thickness burn (*bottom left*); a

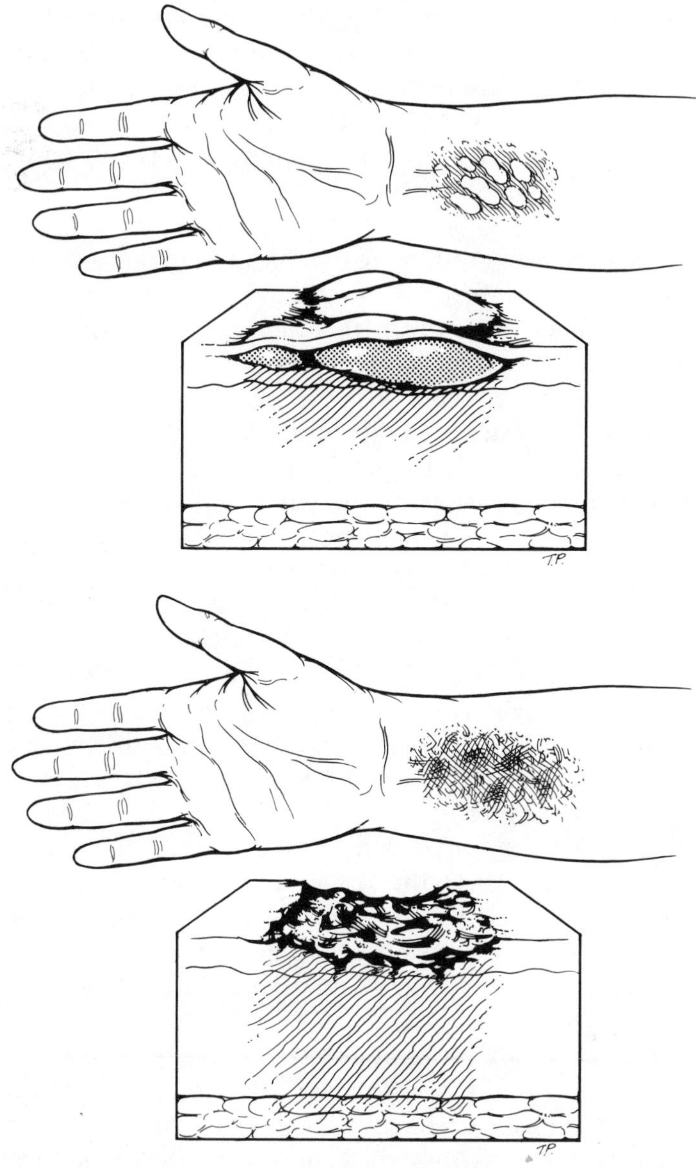

deep partial-thickness burn, or deep second-degree burn (*top right*); and a third-degree burn, also called a full-thickness burn (*bottom right*).

ing for a patient with a second-degree burn, even though the burn might heal on its own. The surgical treatment is intended to reduce scarring: a second-degree burn that takes a long time to heal often heals with a lot of scarring and thickening. Scarring usually can be prevented with an early operation. Surgery is only possible when there is enough donor skin and the patient is fit for surgery, however.

Third-degree burns destroy the full thickness of skin—all of the epidermis and all of the dermis—and are commonly caused by contact with flame or liquids with a high boiling point (fat, tar, molten metal). A third-degree burn appears dry, pale, and leathery. The skin will not grow back. Skin grafts must be performed to keep infection from entering the body through the burn (see below).

Full-thickness burned skin contracts and loses its ability to stretch. It becomes tight around the extremity, eventually restricting the blood supply to the hand or foot or limiting chest expansion during breathing. Third-degree burns that encircle the arm or leg or chest require an *escharotomy*. An escharotomy, usually performed in the emergency room or upon admission to the medical unit or the burn unit, is an incision in the burn made through the skin to the underlying fat. Because third-degree burns destroy nerve endings, the burned skin is numb and anesthesia is generally not needed for this procedure, although some sedation or pain medication may be given.

Fourth-degree burns involve the tissues beneath the skin such as muscle and bone. This term is rarely used, because burns of this depth are rare. They are usually caused by high-voltage electricity or by sleeping close to a fire for a long time in an altered state of consciousness. The limb is often destroyed and amputation is necessary.

There are no reliable scientific tests to judge the depth of the burn or the ability of the wound to heal without skin-grafting procedures. The medical team must inspect and feel the burn and estimate its depth. Generally speaking, second-degree burns blister and hurt more than third degree burns (because some of the skin nerves are still alive), but this is not always true. Quite often, the burn wound "evolves" over several days, particularly in children, and the physician cannot be sure of the depth for quite a while. This explains why it is not unusual for the estimate of the burn depth to change with time and why it is a good idea not to press the physician early on to tell you what he thinks of the burn depth. Sometimes only with the passage of time is it possible to determine the full extent of the injury.

Next: The Treatment Plan

For the first two or three days after the injury, the patient will receive fluids to make up the huge body fluid losses that seep out from the burn (this procedure is called *resuscitation*). The patient may be fed intravenously and may receive mechanical assistance with breathing and circulation (see Chapter 3). The burn wound is cleaned by the staff once or twice a day and then dressed, usually with a medication designed to kill germs (a burn cream) and thick dressings. The treatment of the burn is painful, and the patient will receive pain medications to ease the pain. Management of pain is an essential concern of the medical team, the nursing team, and the rehabilitation team (see below).

Specialists are frequently called in to consult with the doctors directly in charge of the burn patient. These individuals are highly qualified in medical areas such as infection control or the treatment of the various specific organ systems that may fail as a result of the burn. The role of these specialists in helping the medical or burn team manage the patient is described in detail in Chapter 3.

Treatment of the burn wound

The wounds are cleansed once or twice daily with a detergent made up of antiseptic solutions. This cleansing, called *debridement*, is a necessary part of burn wound treatment. Debriding the skin involves removing loose, dead skin and old creams or secretions from the skin.

After debridement, antibiotic cream or solutions are applied directly to the burn. Silvadene, Sulfamylon, Bacitracin, Bibiotic, and silver nitrate are some examples. Sterile dressings are then usually placed over the wounds, although sometimes the wounds are left uncovered. Occasionally special dressings that look like clear plastic or medicated gauze are applied to wounds.

Some medical teams prefer to change dressings and clean

wounds during *hydrotherapy*, using a water tub. This is called "tubbing." Either in the tub or at the bedside, the burns are debrided at least once each day. The family is advised not to visit during or just after a debridement or dressing change. The patient is in pain and the staff is harassed. Wait half an hour after the dressing is finished, or visit before the dressing change takes place.

Treatment of specific types of burns

Some types of burns require additional specific treatment. Chemical burns, for example, are caused by alkalis, acids, oxidants, or other agents that destroy tissue upon contact. Chemical burns need to be rinsed with water to remove all traces of the toxic material. This is best done immediately, and with shower water, but occasionally chemical wounds are also treated with specific antidotes such as calcium injections or applications of an ammonium gel (for hydrofluoric acid burns). The chemical burn wound is then treated like any other burn wound.

A person with a high-voltage electrical burn is treated differently than someone with a flame injury. Electrical injury causes damage to tissues beneath the skin surface: the electrical current passes through the body, heating the bone and causing damage to muscles from the inside out. Blood vessels also become damaged, and delayed muscle death can occur from the lack of circulation over the days to weeks following the initial injury. This internal damage causes swelling that in turn could cause further muscle and nerve injury. To prevent this, early surgery is performed to release pressure on muscle and nerves caused by swollen deep tissues.

For the person with a high-voltage electrical burn, repeated trips to the operating room for debridement are often needed. Once the burn wound is healthy, exposed bone and tendons may need to be covered by *local flaps* (adjacent healthy tissue transferred over the wound) or microvascular *free flaps* (healthy tissue transferred from another part of the body). Amputation of damaged fingers, toes, and even parts of limbs is necessary in up to two-thirds of high-voltage injuries.

Electrical current can cause arrhythmias (irregular heartbeats) or even cardiac arrest (cessation of heartbeat) as well as respiratory arrest (cessation of breathing). Other injuries, such as fractures and head injuries, can result when the body is thrown after receiving the electrical shock. Kidney damage can occur when products are released from damaged muscle cells (myoglobinuria). All of these conditions and injuries must be treated along with the burns themselves.

Flash burns from an electrical accident are similar to flame burns and are managed in the same fashion.

Tar burns cause deep burns because of the high temperatures and prolonged contact with the skin. The tar can be removed with ointments and creams, a procedure that can be done more leisurely if the wound has first been cooled.

What can we expect after two or three days?

If things are going well in the first two or three days, the swelling will decrease, the patient's state of consciousness will improve, blood pressure will stabilize, and, for a patient on the respirator, the oxygen concentration will be decreased. If all of the patient's burns are second-degree burns and the body percentage involved is moderate, the patient is now usually mobilized (see Chapter 4) and discharge planning may begin.

The oxygen content of the air the patient is receiving via respirator or face mask is one indication of the patient's progress. Ask the physician or nurse *what percent oxygen* the patient is breathing. The oxygen content of air is 21 percent, so if the patient is receiving air with an oxygen content close to that—say, 30 to 35 percent oxygen—the patient is nearing the point where the breathing tube can be removed. If the patient's lungs were badly injured by smoke inhalation, the degree of support given by the respirator will increase rather than decrease as time goes on. It is not a good sign if a patient's oxygen content is increased from 50 up to 60 percent, for example. The percent of inspired or breathed oxygen is referred to as the FIO_2 (ef-i-oh-two) in medical jargon.

Early kidney failure is unusual, but very old people do sometimes experience kidney failure early on. People with very deep burns and with high-voltage electrical burns also sometimes have early kidney failure. It is usually reversible, but artificial kidney treatment (*dialysis*) is sometimes required. Milder forms of kidney failure due to burn shock are common and usually are of little consequence.

How long will it take for the burns to heal?

It depends on the depth of the burn and the patient's age, overall health, and nutritional status. First-degree burns fade and become pain free within one week. Second-degree or superficial partial-thickness burns heal in two to three weeks, although deeper burns can take four to five weeks. Third-degree burns need to be excised or removed surgically and then covered by skin grafts from an unburned area of the body or with the patient's cultured skin (see below).

Special Problems

Infection

Infection, or *sepsis*, is the enemy of burn patients. Sepsis is not usually a threat within the first few days after the injury, but it becomes a serious threat after the first week. One of the most difficult and frustrating things for a family to understand is that a patient who does extraordinarily well during the first two or three days after major burn injury can become extremely ill—indeed, can succumb—several weeks after admission, just when things seem to be going well.

The truth is that no patient with a major burn is safe from the complication of sepsis until the burn wound is completely grafted or has healed, all intravenous lines have been removed and the patient is eating, all antibiotics have been discontinued, and the patient has no fever for several days.

Infection occurs when bacteria or germs enter the burn wound and the tissues surrounding it. Bacteria come from the air, from the patient's own skin, or through the medical tubes or any other source of external contamination. They may come from inside the patient's body, such as from the bowel or intestines, where bacteria normally live quietly, causing no harm. Dead tissue from the burn acts as a medium for bacterial growth; that is, it provides a fertile place for bacteria to grow in. Dead tissue also has a poor blood supply. This means that antibiotics, which are administered through the bloodstream, have difficulty reaching the burn wound and therefore bacteria are able to multiply despite treatment with antibiotics.

A burn patient's natural defense mechanisms against infection are depleted, and infections can advance rapidly and become quite serious in a short period of time. Burn wound sepsis can destroy living tissue, changing or "converting" the wound to a deeper injury, such as from a superficial to a deep partial-thickness burn, or from a second-degree to a third-degree burn. Burn patients who develop infection are at serious risk.

Samples of blood, urine, and sputum and biopsies of the burn wound itself are obtained as cultures to determine the presence and type of bacteria. Fever is another indication of infection which can be measured. Infection is treated with topical (applied on the wound) and systemic (given intravenously) antibiotics. A further treatment, performed when the patient is stable, is the surgical removal of dead skin and underlying tissue—called *excision* of the wound.

Pain

All burn patients experience pain, and it can be excruciating. For the family and friends of burn patients, witnessing the pain of a loved one is heartbreaking. The staff of the medical center or burn center must cope with the patient's pain, too. Pain is something that must be worked through with courage and determination by all.

The injury is painful because nerve endings are exposed when the skin is burned away. In addition, when skin grafting is performed (see below), the donor site is also painful. Pain can be alleviated, but it is not abolished until the burn is healed. Aside from general anesthesia, no pain medication will completely remove a patient's pain. Nevertheless, controlling the patient's pain is one of the medical team's most important tasks.

The patient's comfort is important psychologically for both the patient and the family. Pain medications may be prescribed to allow the patient to sleep, to provide the patient respite from agitation, or to calm the patient down. This is crucial, since burn patients are often anxious, and anxiety can increase pain. Burn patients may be anxious because they feel they are being punished for their real or imagined involvement in the cause of their burn injury, or they may be afraid of the treatments they face each day or of what lies ahead (see Chapter 5 for a discussion of these issues).

Medications are also used to treat the delirium and depression that frequently occur after major burn injuries.

Pain control is important not only for the patient's comfort but also for the patient's recovery. Pain medications that "take the edge off" the pain also make the pain bearable for the patient so that wounds can be treated properly during dressing changes and tub baths. Pain medications enable the patient in rehabilitation to cooperate with physical therapy and perform range-of-motion exercises to regain the strength and mobility lost during hospitalization. And pain medication helps the patient get the rest and sleep he or she needs to recover properly.

It is often difficult for patients and families to accept the fact that pain medicines cannot be administered all the time or at very high doses all the time. But pain medications are serious and sometimes dangerous drugs that must be administered by an experienced person who uses good judgment in balancing the patient's need for pain control with the patient's other needs—pain medications cannot be given in such large doses that they interfere with the function of the patient's internal organs, for example. And pain medications must be given at prescribed intervals so the patient does not become dependent on them or develop side effects. When you hear a nurse or a doctor say to a patient, "It's not time for your pain medicine yet," you can be reasonably certain that the nurse or doctor has the patient's best interests in mind.

Sometimes relaxation techniques such as hypnosis or creative imagery are used to help control pain. In creative imagery, the nurse, social worker, or psychologist talks to the patient and takes the patient mentally to another place. For example, the patient can be asked to imagine that he or she is visiting a favorite vacation spot. This process helps the patient focus on something other than the pain. It can create a safe haven to harbor the patient while he or she rides the waves of pain. Listening to music, practicing deep breathing, and focusing visually on a pleasant object are other relaxation techniques that are effective for some people.

Children react to pain in a variety of ways. Younger children may scream, cry, kick, and even withdraw. Most frequently they'll show a lack of interest in play and other pleasurable activities. Children who are older can talk about their pain, but they too may exhibit aggressive behaviors as an expression of their pain. When children of all ages experience pain, they may take their anger and frustration out on family members or health care professionals who participate in their care.

Children in pain require very special treatment. First, the staff can make certain the child is given the proper pain medication on the proper schedule. Staff members and families can give reassurance and listen attentively to the child's concerns. Children deserve and benefit from clear and honest explanations of all the treatments they receive. When possible, all procedures should be administered in a designated treatment room, away from the child's usual environment (bedroom and play areas). This allows the child to have a safe environment where he or she knows painful procedures won't occur.

A variety of methods can be used to help the child focus on something other than the pain. Distraction can be especially effective with younger children. Playing with toys, listening to music and singing, talking quietly, and focusing on an object in the room can provide distraction for the child. Relaxation techniques such as those described above can assist the child through painful procedures and other unpleasant experiences.

Having a feeling of control over unpleasant procedures may aid in reducing the child's pain. Allowing the child to remove old dressings, make decisions about the order in which procedures will be performed, and set time limits for procedures will help comfort the child. Families and staff members need to listen attentively and provide feedback. Children—no less than adults—need to know that they are being heard.

Step Four: Skin Grafting

If the patient has deep second-degree burns or third-degree burns, the health care team begins to make plans for the next step—surgery—once the patient is stable and a treatment plan has been drawn up. Surgery is an essential part of the treatment plan for all patients with third-degree burns and for some patients with second-degree burns. The burn wounds must be covered with new skin both to prevent infection and to limit scarring, which may interfere with the person's ability to function.

The principal surgical operation performed on burn patients is skin grafting. In this procedure, a sliver of the patient's skin is removed from a healthy, unburned area (the *donor area*) and attached to the area destroyed by the burn (the *recipient area*) by stitches, staples, or adhesive paper strips or simply by dressings. Before receiving the donor skin, the recipient area must be prepared to accept the donor skin. This may be done either surgically, by excision, or by allowing the heat-damaged skin (the *eschar*) to separate naturally from the underlying, healthy tissue.

Excision is performed on the areas of the burn that have not or are not expected to heal on their own, that is, the deep second-degree and third-degree full-thickness burn. It is often used for extensive third-degree burns of a large surface area and burns of an entire extremity.

In excision, the eschar is removed either tangentially or fascially. *Tangential* excision involves removing the eschar with a long razor blade in layers until all dead tissue is gone and the surface consists of healthy tissue. This usually is the deepest layer of dermis or the fat beneath the dermis (subcutaneous fat). This technique preserves the maximum amount of viable tissue. Excision *down to fascia* involves removing the entire layer of damaged skin and underlying fat down to the fascia—the tough covering over the underlying muscle—all at once. This is a quick way of removing large amounts of burned skin with less blood loss than occurs with tangential excision. A healthier grafting surface is also achieved with excision down to fascia.

Excision usually promotes early healing and eliminates a source of infection. Despite its advantages, this technique is sometimes used reluctantly because the final appearance after removal of fat can be less pleasing. Another disadvantage of excision is the inevitability of blood loss, making transfusions the rule, not the exception. When excision is performed, there is also usually a need for prolonged or multiple anesthesias.

Sometimes the eschar is allowed to fall off without surgery, by natural separation. As the eschar lifts off the wound, it is gradually removed or debrided during dressing changes and tubbings. This method decreases the need for anesthetics and is less traumatic to underlying, healthy tissue than excision. But there are disadvantages to this method, too. Natural separation of the eschar takes three to five weeks and therefore involves a delay in closing the wound, prolonged hospitalization, and an increased risk of infection. This method is often used for areas such as the face, to conserve viable tissue, and the palms and soles, where the skin is thick. It is also used when the patient is medically ill or the depth of the burn cannot be determined.

Once the eschar is removed, if there is not enough remaining dermis, which contains regenerating elements (epidermal cells in hair follicles and sweat glands), new skin will not grow. Skin must be transferred from an unburned part of the body. The patient donates his own skin (autograft) in a surgical procedure in which the surgeon removes skin from unburned areas. Only a partial layer of skin is removed from the donor site, so that the dermis that remains on the donor site will generate new epidermis. Donor areas can be any part of the body, but since they heal with scarring, inconspicuous areas are used first if possible. Common sites include the thigh, abdomen, trunk, and even the scalp (which must be shaved before surgery begins).

The donor sites are like new partial-thickness burns and are treated as such, with gauze dressings (dry or medicated, such as Xeriform and Scarlet Red) or plastic dressings (Opsite, Tegaderm, and others) or synthetic gauzes (Biobrane). These donor sites are like second-degree burns in other ways, too: they are subject to pain, scarring, and infection, and they must be protected. Donor site healing is usually complete within 7 to 10 days. Once the donor site has healed, new skin grafts can be obtained or "harvested" from the same area.

The skin from the donor site may be stretched to allow it to cover a larger area than it came from, a procedure called *meshing*. This involves making small slits in the skin which allow it to expand like fish netting (Figure 1.3). Meshing serves two purposes: it allows blood and body fluids to drain from under the skin grafts (accumulated fluids interfere with healing), and it allows the skin to stretch over a greater area. Meshing works very well, but on widely "meshed" skin the mesh marks may be visible forever on the healed burn.

Multiple trips to the operating room are often required before all the eschar is removed and the entire burn wound is grafted. The length of hospitalization is quite variable and depends to a large

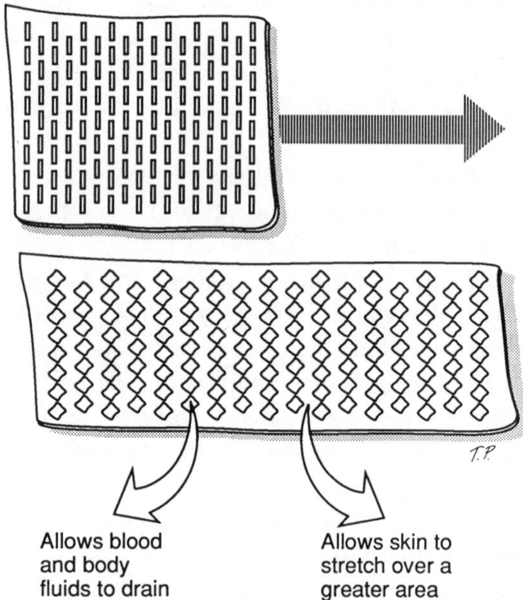

Figure 1.3. Meshed skin grafts allow blood and body fluids to drain from under the skin grafts and allow the skin to stretch over a greater area.

degree on the patient's condition and on any complications that occur. It is not unusual for a patient with major burns to be hospitalized for six to eight weeks or more.

Skin and skin substitutes

When the burn wound covers a large area, the available donor areas may not provide enough skin to cover the entire excised wound. Sometimes, too, the patient is not healthy enough to tolerate a prolonged operation or the harvesting of more skin. And sometimes cultured skin has been ordered but is not expected to be available for several weeks. In these situations, many temporary coverings may be used until the patient's own skin or cultured skin is available. The following types of skin and skin substitutes are available:

Autograft. This is the patient's own skin, as described above.

Allograft or homograft. This is human skin donated from a deceased person which is stored, or banked, after undergoing rigorous testing for transmittable disease. Tissue banks adhere to the standards of the American Association of Tissue Banks. These standards state that the donor's medical history must be screened and the donor tested for HIV (the virus that causes AIDS) and hepatitis virus. The skin is not released until these results are known to be negative. The skin is frozen and stored at –80°C; this provides additional protection against contaminants.

Allografts are applied and managed just like the patient's own grafted skin (autograft). Eventually allografts will be rejected by the patient's immune system, but before this they will actually adhere to the wound as in the normal healing process. Allografts keep the wound closed until donor sites have healed sufficiently to allow reharvesting or until cultured skin is available.

Skin replacement research is ongoing, and every year brings more advances. Initial experimental success has been reported in a handful of patients around the world who have had permanent allograft transplants and have taken the immunosuppressive drug cyclosporine to prevent rejection of the donor skin. This procedure is in its infancy, however, and its value has not been proven. Some doctors are now trying to use homograft for the deep or dermal portion of the replaced skin, and cultured skin (see below) for the more superficial or epidermal portion. As this book is being written, this is a very promising technique.

Cultured skin. Cultured skin, or cultured autograft, is a relatively new method of healing the wound and is used when the patient's own available skin graft donor sites are insufficient. Burn wounds are excised as usual, and the site is covered with allograft or other biologic dressings until sufficient cultured skin is available.

To produce cultured autograft, a tiny piece of skin is taken from an unburned area of the patient's body and its cells are grown in layers in laboratory petri dishes. The skin grows in small sheets that are then applied to the burn. This method expands the patient's own epidermis from a 1-inch sample up to more than 250 yards of skin—a 10,000-fold increase—over a 30-day period.

The advantages of cultured skin are that the biopsy site is very small and the skin is the patient's "own," so it isn't rejected. The disadvantages? Cultured skin takes three weeks to grow, it is quite fragile, and it is very expensive. Healed cultured skin is often very fragile, too; it is easily damaged and is subject to blistering, since there is no underlying layer of dermis, but only epidermis covering the tissues beneath.

Artificial skin. There is no complete, permanent, true artificial skin yet, although work on artificial dermis is in progress. It is hoped that artificial skin will allow earlier coverage of the burn wound independent of donor site healing; this would lead to shorter hospital stays and improved survival of the severely burned patient.

There are many good temporary artificial wound coverings. All of them eventually must be replaced with autograft. The best of the artificial skins developed so far is a two-layered product, the inside layer being biologic (this stays on the patient) and the outside being plastic (this part is replaced by autograft). The autograft replacing the plastic is much thinner than conventional autograft, so that the donor site heals in 3 to 5 days instead of 7 to 10 days, which is a great advantage.

Animal skin and human fetal membranes. Commercially processed pigskin and human fetal membranes are used by some surgeons as a temporary covering for the burn wound. Closing wounds with these dressings has the advantages of reducing the loss of protein fluid and electrolytes from the wound, decreasing pain in the wound, and facilitating the healing of partial-thickness burns. Furthermore, if the biologic dressing becomes adherent, it is a sign that the wound is ready to support an autograft.

It should be emphasized that none of these skin substitutes is like buying aspirin off the shelf—using them takes experience and skill. Patients who have these procedures *must* be in the hands of experienced burn surgeons.

What happens after skin grafting?

Grafts, whether they are auto or allo, are either left open to the air or are wrapped in dressings, sometimes with antibiotic solutions or creams applied. "Take down" is the first dressing change after the grafting procedure and occurs usually two to five days after the procedure. At this point the "take"—the amount of the graft that is viable and adherent—is estimated.

The take is often expressed as a percentage of the grafted area. A take of more than 85 percent means the procedure was a success. Not all of the skin graft needs to take in order for the wound to completely heal, since small open areas can heal in from the surrounding edges. If the take is less than 60 percent, another patching procedure usually must be performed. Infection, movement, and complications can interfere with the take rate.

Grafted areas need to be protected from rubbing by clothing or activity, especially early after grafting. The healed or grafted skin may also be itchy and dry. Frequent application of moisturizers—ideally lotions that have a water-soluble base—such as lanolin and Eucerin will help decrease dryness and itching. Itching is caused by the chemicals that are released in the wound during the healing process. Dryness results from the absence of normal oil glands in the split-thickness skin graft.

If there is need for further grafting, the surgery is repeated until the wound is covered with new skin. Once the burn wound is healed, there is less and less need for dressings, until the newly healed or grafted areas can be left totally open. Many patients are discharged from the hospital while still requiring dressings.

Grafted skin will always look different from normal skin, although many aspects can be changed with surgery and also with the passage of time. Healed skin grafts often are redder or darker than surrounding skin and have irregular raised areas. Skin that has healed by itself or with skin grafting is less sensitive to touch and will always be somewhat more easily damaged than normal skin.

If the grafting was successful, can anything else go wrong?

Unfortunately, yes. We go day by day, rejoicing as progress is made but never becoming totally confident. A burn patient is cured only when he or she is out of the hospital, heading home. We have already discussed lung failure (usually from smoke inhalation), kidney failure, and infection. All of these, particularly infection, can occur after a promising, uncomplicated first few days. In older people, particularly those with a history of heart or blood pressure problems, the heart or circulation can fail. Burn patients sometimes develop stomach ulcers and other abdominal problems, although these are rare.

The burn team is experienced in discovering these complications and acting to treat them very quickly. No news is good news: if the family hears nothing about unexpected developments, the family can assume that everything is going well.

Going Home

The length of stay in the hospital can be as short as a few hours or as long as many months. The average length of stay in U.S. hospitals is 14 days. It is sometimes estimated that if there are no complications, the patient will be in the hospital one day for every percentage point of the body surface that is burned. But such an estimate can only be approximate, and the person's age, overall health, and other factors also affect the length of the hospital stay.

In most cases discharge planning will begin soon after the grafting procedures end, and the patient is set upon the long course to recovery. It is most important that family members and friends stay mentally and physically fit to help with the recovery process. Long nightly vigils in the hospital during the acute illness are to be discouraged: they don't help the patient and they lead to exhaustion for the family. Time will come when the patient will require the full vigor of support of family and friends: let us save our strength.

Along the same lines, although it is difficult to advise families about their behavior that is not strictly relevant to patient care, it is important that family and friends try to live their lives as normally as possible while the patient is in the hospital. Family members are frequently under the impression that the staff (or the patient) expects them to sit around night and day to be available. Although the presence of loved ones is critical to recovery, family members also need to do what is necessary for them to stay mentally and physically healthy through what may become a prolonged period of stress.

Chapter 2

Family and Friends

A trauma such as a burn injury has a profound impact not only on the injured person but on everyone involved in this person's life, including parents, siblings, spouses, children, friends, and co-workers. As the patient fights for life, family members are dealing with the shock and chaos that has entered their lives. What once seemed so important, like vacation plans, becomes trivial in the face of death. Normal routines have been replaced with long hours at the hospital, last-minute child care arrangements, and extended visits by well-meaning family and friends. Nothing is as it was.

The medical unit's social worker, counselor, or staff psychologist, each of whom is trained in crisis intervention, can be helpful to the family throughout this ordeal. The family's needs must be addressed along with the needs of the patient, for the family will eventually become the primary caregivers and will assume responsibility for the patient's day-to-day care. If the family's needs are continually ignored, the family may become overwhelmed and be unable to perform the role of caregivers.

The purpose of this chapter is to provide support for the families and friends of burn survivors and to help them understand their role in the burn survivor's recovery. In this chapter, the hospital stay is divided into three phases: the survival phase, the functional phase, and the visual phase. It's important to keep in mind, though, that each person is unique and that these phases will be different for various individuals. Any of the issues described as surfacing during a particular phase may arise in another—or be apparent during all three phases simultaneously. The phases themselves overlap: they are presented here as distinct phases only for purposes of clarity.

The Survival Phase

In the early days and weeks following injury, the patient's condition may be critical, and the possibility of death may loom large. The medical treatment of the patient in these early weeks is aggressive, with daily dressing changes, fluid and antibiotic therapies, and surgical interventions. Often the patient is on a respirator or is too sick to communicate with the staff and family. Not being able to talk with the patient is difficult for family members, who are trying to come to terms with the possibility that their loved one may die.

The family looks to the staff for guidance and reassurance, but there are no guarantees. Staff members are guarded when talking with the family, careful not to give false hope. Every sentence begins with "if," "maybe," or "in time." These statements become sources of frustration and perhaps anger for family members, who are naturally looking for more definite answers. But medicine is not an exact science.

The family struggles to remain hopeful despite uncertainties or a poor prognosis. As the days drag on, they begin to realize and accept the gravity of the situation. The grieving process has begun, as evidenced by their acceptance of a possible poor outcome. The family needs to mourn their losses both actual (change in lifestyle) and potential (death of the patient). Staff members are aware of this mourning process and generally allow the family the opportunity to express their feelings without fear of rejection or judgment.

The emotions the family experiences in this stage will run the gamut from anxiety and fear to despair and depression. Family members may feel as if they're drowning in a flood of emotions. They often feel as if they are going "crazy" if they can't stop crying, if they feel numb, or if they are angry with the patient for getting injured. All of these feelings and emotions are normal under the circumstances. Again, it is best if the family feels comfortable expressing these emotions, because if they are left unaddressed, they could result in significant harm to the family and the patient.

Another prominent emotion is helplessness. The staff is providing the patient with everything he or she needs, leaving little for the family to do in terms of physical care. Usually the staff will try to get the family involved by explaining the function of the numerous machines and monitors and by describing the purpose of the various procedures performed. Information is the family's only weapon against feeling completely useless. The more the family learns about burns and burn care, the better equipped they will be to assist their loved one in the recovery process. Family support has been shown to increase significantly the positive outcome for the severely burn-injured patient.

Clearly, the first priority of staff members is the patient. From time to time the staff may become impatient with the family's questions and demands for information. If this becomes an issue, the unit social worker or counselor will generally intervene and establish a specific time for the family to meet with members of the medical team to discuss the patient's condition and treatment. We encourage family members to bring a list of questions to this meeting and to take notes during the meeting. Writing down explanations and asking the nurses and doctors to repeat or thoroughly explain the information will help the family better understand the information relayed and prevent misunderstanding when the information is conveyed to other family members. This is also an excellent opportunity for the medical team to learn about the patient's preburn functioning, personality, and coping styles. This information will be very useful to the therapists who develop the patient's treatment plan.

Questions about quality of life often arise. When the patient is too sick or confused to contribute to the discussion meaningfully and let his or her wishes be known, the family must make decisions for the patient. This is where the family must think things through and determine what they think the *patient* would wish, and what *they* would wish for the patient. Doctors must obey the law and ethical and moral guidelines, but beyond that, the input of the family and friends is vitally important when the patient is not able to make decisions about treatment. If a severely injured person has executed a living will or has issued a power of attorney covering treatment or any aspect of life support, this document must immediately be brought to the attention of the treatment team.

No two people respond the same way to stress, even if they are related. So it is likely that as the crisis moves into a more permanent state, the different coping styles of different family members will emerge. Incompatible coping styles may be a major source of misunderstanding between family members, especially when anxiety levels are high. Anxiety can cloud judgment, and behavior can easily be misunderstood.

For example, suppose that a mother seeks out information from the staff at every opportunity, is constantly at the child's bedside, and participates in the dressing changes. In contrast, the child's father spends most of his time in the lobby, rarely speaks with the staff, and observes procedures from a distance. The wife may interpret her husband's behavior as representing a lack of love for the child or for herself. Believing she can no longer rely on her husband, she turns once again to the staff or other family members for support. Her husband, meanwhile, interprets her close relationship with the staff as another insult to his ability to provide for and protect his family. The pain this couple is feeling prevents them from seeing the real meaning behind their behavior. Neither of them will be able to support the other until both of them understand that their behavior is not indicative of serious differences but represents the playing out of their opposite coping styles. The wife needs to recognize that her husband's distance is a sign not that he doesn't care but that he is unable to watch his child in pain. The husband must learn to accept the fact that he can't do it all and that it's okay to get help from others. This couple's behavior illustrates how anxiety and stress can impede a family's functioning.

This phase encompasses the initial crisis following the injury and the interventions made to assist the family with their shock. The relationships established early between the family and the staff will be invaluable later, as the patient's condition improves and she becomes an active participant in her treatment.

What if the patient is in a coma?

One question that medical science has not yet been able to answer is the question of how much a person who is in a coma or is heavily sedated can feel or hear. Even though the burn team doesn't know whether the patient can hear them, they always behave as if the patient understands every word spoken in his presence, and it is a good idea for family members and other visitors to behave this way, too. In fact, starting with the assumption that sedated patients can hear and understand what is said, visitors are encouraged to bring the patient interesting news from home and the outside world, to keep him engaged in what is going on around him.

The Functional Phase

In this phase, although death remains a possibility, it is no longer the major focus. Unlike during the acute phase, medical interventions at this time are no longer solely for survival purposes. Most of the efforts are now geared to helping the patient reach his or her maximum functioning potential. Discussions are no longer prefaced with "If the patient gets through the night" or "In time, if the patient . . ." Staff members are less guarded against giving false hope, and a more optimistic tone can be noticed in conversations. This helps to alleviate some of the feeling of crisis and to reduce tension for the family.

The patient has now improved to the point where he can actively participate in his own care. With the increasing comfort, however, come new challenges: the rapidity with which changes take place can be frightening for both the patient and the family. Family and friends may find it difficult to keep up with the constant transitions. The staff will continue to help the family remain informed about treatments and therapies. Family members are encouraged to continue preparing questions ahead of time and to write down information as it is obtained. As this phase progresses, new information will be introduced quite rapidly; this information will be essential during the patient's rehabilitation.

As the patient's condition stabilizes and shows signs of improvement, the family will begin to relax and may even begin thinking in terms of the future. The family now needs to regain some control in their lives and begin to resume some of their normal activities: work, banking, laundry, school, and so on. The family may consider staying away from the hospital for a day so they can take care of other matters, or perhaps they'll want to leave before visiting hours are over. This is the start of the natural separation process. The patient may see this as abandonment and begin to play on the family's emotions, trying to make them feel guilty. The family can help by pointing out to their loved one how important it is for the patient to do things independently and gently reminding him how much he hated being dependent on others to brush his teeth or wash his face. The more independent the patient becomes, the sooner he will be able to go home. This time can be used by the family as respite, because once the patient is home, there will be little leisure time.

The patient may be only just beginning to realize the severity of the injury, whereas the family has had days or in some cases weeks to deal with the shock and begin to cope with the situation. This discrepancy—between the *patient's* psychological state and where the *family* has progressed psychologically—will create difficulty. The patient needs time to catch up on all that she has missed. The patient needs to be educated about burns, for example. The patient also needs to have the opportunity to mourn for her losses (lifestyle, job, and so on), just as the family did in the beginning. The patient cannot fully appreciate how close to death she came. To the patient, the idea of total or even partial dependence on others is devastating.

In the family's vew, the patient has greatly improved from those "early days" when he wasn't even able to breathe for himself. The family may try to help by saying things like "But you look so much better" or "But last week you couldn't even open your eyes." The family's intentions are good, but the effect may be to create bigger problems. If the patient is encouraged to ignore these intense feelings, the patient may begin to "act out" on the unit (usually by becoming aggressive) or become depressed, refusing to participate in therapy. Everyone—staff and family—needs to remember how important it is for the injured individual to express his feelings without fear of reprisal or judgment, just as it was for the family.

The family may try to quiet the patient as a way of avoiding the rehashing of such horrible memories, because they want to spare the patient the pain *they* went through. This is normal, as is wanting to forget and put this tragedy behind them. However, the patient needs to address some issues before going on. The family and the social worker or counselor can work together to help the patient gradually adjust in his or her own way. As the family focuses their energies elsewhere, the patient is given time to come to terms with the injury. The patient will either accept the situation and work on getting better or deny it and resist doing what is necessary for improvement. The latter attitude can be an extremely frustrating one for family members, who can only sit and watch this unfold.

In this phase the rehabilitation team makes a comprehensive assessment of what the patient can and can't do. Armed with this information, they establish a personalized treatment plan that will maximize strengths while addressing weaknesses. Patients may undergo physical and occupational therapy for more than three hours a day. They work on feeding and dressing themselves and on walking. For the recovering burn patient, confronting limitations and a new appearance can be horrifying. The information provided by the family to the staff in the early weeks will be used at this time to challenge and motivate the patient.

As the patient prepares for the day of discharge, so too must the family. Special arrangements need to be made for the care of young children, and medical equipment such as a walker, a commode chair, and dressing supplies need to be ordered. Furniture may need to be rearranged from various floors or rooms. A home care agency might become involved to assist with wound care and physical therapy at home. All of this is coordinated with the social worker or discharge planner, who will sit down with the family as discharge nears and discuss at length the patient's needs, the family's resources, and any issues not yet addressed. The nurses start teaching the family how to bathe or shower the patient, care for wounds, and do other things. They will tell the family about the patient's needs in terms of medicines and diet. The therapists will also instruct the family in the home exercise program that will be performed between therapy sessions.

As you can see, this phase is packed with movement and new information. It is essential that families be actively involved in these preparations. Otherwise the patient's discharge could be a traumatic experience instead of a triumph. As all of these arrangements are being made, the patient and the family are moving into the third and final phase, visibility.

The Visual Phase

Now that the threat of death is remote and the patient's functioning abilities are known, the reality of the patient's altered appearance weighs heavily on all. The patient is no longer confined to the burn unit; he or she is free to move about the hospital visiting the cafeteria, the gift shop, the rehabilitation department. During these excursions off the unit the patient will encounter many people who have never seen a burn injury. These persons may stare at or even mock the patient. Curious people may approach the patient and ask questions, some of which may be quite inappropriate. Since this appearance is new to the patient as well, he or she may not be prepared to deal with these encounters.

If the patient becomes angry and has never learned how to diffuse that anger, a fight may ensue. Or perhaps the patient will become overwhelmed and start crying uncontrollably. Still another response may be denial—pretending that the situation never occurred. Any of these reactions is likely to occur if the patient is not properly prepared. The patient can not be protected from the world beyond the safety of the burn unit, but with professional help he or she can learn the skills needed to deal with these situations and will able to reenter society. (For more on this and other coping strategies, see chapter 5.)

The patient will still become angry, overwhelmed, or depressed. This is expected. But with professional intervention the fallout from these emotions can be minimized, limiting the damage from traumatic social experiences. Families, too, must learn to cope with these reactions from society. Again, the social worker or counselor will teach the family coping techniques.

The society in which we live can be painfully cruel to anything or anyone that is different from the norm. We fear what we don't understand. The unknown or the unexplained frustrates many people to the point of paralysis. Burn survivors and their families will become all too familiar with this truth.

The patient will be aggressively working with the social worker or counselor to adjust to his or her appearance, which may change several times over the course of many months. The family may be overlooked during this process, because, unlike the patient, they do not carry with them the visible signs of burn injury. Yet the family, like the patient, remembers the patient's preburn appearance. They are struggling to integrate the new appearance into their psychological memory of the patient.

Just as the patient may hope this appearance is temporary, so too might the family. They may bring in pictures of the patient taken before the burn to show to the staff. Or they may place unrealistic expectations on plastic surgery, believing the patient will look the same as before the burn. It is difficult for the family to accept that this injury has changed the patient forever.

The family is encouraged to talk about these expectations as a way of working through this struggle. Admitting they want the patient to look like he or she looked before is a big step in eventually letting go of the old image and accepting the patient's new image.

Many burn survivors believe that before they can accept their appearance and go on with their lives, they must first forget what they used to look like. In a sense they must say good-bye to their old appearance, the one they were born with, and start over, creating a new identity for themselves. Since our identities are closely connected with our appearance, one can see how difficult a task this integration of preburn and postburn appearance can be. The family requires as much assistance dealing with this as does the patient. In time, given appropriate guidance, the family will come to accept the situation and can then begin picking up the pieces of their lives. The family and the patient will start with a clean slate, but the memories of this traumatic injury will be forever a part of them and their history.

Chapter 3

Medical Personnel, Procedures, and Equipment

Who are all these physicians taking care of me, and why are there so many of them? What do all these machines do, and how long will they be attached to me? How long will I have to stay in the hospital? *When can I go home?*

Burn patients and their families have many questions about the patient's treatment program, about the medical specialists and other personnel who are making decisions regarding the patient's medical care, about hospital procedures, and about what the future holds. This chapter is designed to answer some of these common questions. In this chapter you'll learn more about the burn unit and the members of the medical team or burn team as well as the devices they employ in treating patients injured by burns.

The Burn Unit

Many hospitals have established specialized units, informally called *burn units*, for the treatment of burn patients who must be hospitalized. A burn unit is usually a separate area of the hospital which is dedicated to the treatment of patients with burn injuries. The burn unit is equipped with the specialized technology and supplies used in monitoring and treating burn patients. And the staff of the burn unit consists of specialists who devote most of their professional lives to the care of patients whose primary problem is serious burn injury and complications from that injury. The patient in a burn unit will receive a level of care not usually available to someone in a general medical ward of a hospital.

While the burn unit is a separate unit of the hospital, in almost all cases it is still part of the hospital and shares many facilities with the rest of the hospital. (The Shriners Burns Institutes of Boston, Cincinnati, and Galveston, which are freestanding, university-affiliated burn hospitals, are exceptions to this rule.) The facilities the burn unit shares with the hospital include laboratories for blood tests and radiologic examinations (x-ray, computerized tomography scans, and magnetic resonance imaging), the food service, and the operating room.

A patient in the burn unit may have to wait to use the facilities of the hospital because the needs of another patient in the hospital are more urgent. For example, a scheduled operation on a burn patient may be delayed or even canceled when another patient needs emergency surgery. When something like this happens, it is difficult for the patient, the patient's family, and the patient's physician. But it may help to keep in mind that there are only so many facilities in the hospital and other patients in the hospital are waiting, too.

Some burn units are small, containing 4 or 6 beds, and others are large, having 20 or more beds. Burn units are usually divided into two sections: an *intensive care unit* (ICU) and a *step-down section.* A person who is critically ill will be treated in the intensive care unit. Here, the ratio of nurses to patients is much higher, both day and night, than in the step-down section, so the injured person can be constantly monitored and can receive frequent treatment—can even be treated continuously, if necessary. When the patient's condition improves, the patient is moved to the step-down section. A patient who is able to feed himself without help or get out of bed on his own, and whose dressings do not need to be changed as frequently, may be moved to the step-down area. Being moved from the intensive care section of the burn unit to the step-down section may be considered a sign of good recovery from burn injury.

When the staff in a burn unit not only treat patients but also engage in teaching and research, the burn unit is called a burn center, and it is usually affiliated with a major institution such as a university. Many people with burn injury are treated successfully and well at a community or general hospital having a burn unit, while some patients will probably fare better in a burn center. For guidance in selecting a burn unit or burn center, consult the official listings of the American Burn Association in Appendix B.

Physician Specialists

Patients in a burn unit come into contact with a variety of physicians who play different roles in their treatment. This variety can be confusing to patients and their families, but they should be reassured to know that all the different physicians they see are important to their recovery. The section that follows describes the physicians who care for burn patients as well as their specific place on the burn team.

The attending physician and the medical director

The final responsibility for planning and coordinating every patient's care belongs to a senior physician called the *attending*. In most areas of the United States, the law requires that every patient in a hospital be assigned an attending physician. When a decision needs to be made about a patient's treatment, whether it be a change in medications or a recommended diagnostic test, the attending physician must be consulted. By carefully monitoring and coordinating the care provided by the many professionals on the burn team, the attending physician makes certain that no effort on the patient's behalf is neglected—and that no effort is dangerously duplicated. In short, the attending physician is medically and legally responsible for the patient's care.

In most burn units in the United States, the attending physician is either a general surgeon or a plastic surgeon; sometimes the attending is an intensivist (a physician who specializes in intensive care). Not so elsewhere in the world, where anesthesiologists, internists (physicians who specialize in the medical, rather than the surgical, treatment of illness), and dermatologists may be the specialists who are in charge of burn units.

The *medical director* of the burn unit has overall administrative responsibility for the unit. He or she must ensure that the unit is fully staffed and equipped to care for the patients in the unit. In some burn units, the medical director is also the attending physician. In a large unit, the responsibility for the care of patients is shared by the medical director and several attending physicians. In this case, too, each patient is usually assigned only one principal attending physician.

Patients in a burn unit and their families and friends should know who the patient's attending physician is, and they should know how to contact the attending. If they are not told how to contact the attending, they should ask a member of the staff how to do so. If they are confused about their treatment or about hospital procedures, or if they have questions that haven't been adequately answered, patients and their families should contact the attending.

Working under the direction of the attending are the fellows, the residents, and the interns.

Fellows, residents, and interns

The *fellow* is a recent graduate of medical school who either has not quite finished surgical training or has finished surgical training but wants to obtain additional experience. Fellows are highly trained and skilled physicians who are polishing or honing their skills. Fellows in the burn unit are working in the unit to improve their knowledge about burn care and their skills in treating burns.

Fellows see each patient in the burn unit frequently during the day, and they direct the resident physicians' day-to-day care of the patient. When their hospital responsibilities end each day, the fellows may return home, but they may be called back to the hospital if a patient develops a problem requiring their attention.

The *residents* and the *interns*, like the fellows, are recent graduates of medical school who are receiving additional training, usually in surgery, and who are "rotating" through the burn service for a month or two. The resident has been out of medical school for two or more years; the intern is in his or her first year postgraduation. The resident or intern writes the daily orders, including orders for pain medications, and takes care of the tubes, or lines, which are attached to the patients (see below).

The residents and interns are the unsung heroes of burn care. They stay in the hospital all night (to say that they sleep is misleading, because they seldom have a chance to catch more than an hour or two of shuteye).

Other specialists

Although the physicians described above are experts in the day-to-day care of the patients in the burn unit and can handle most of the emergencies that arise, occasionally there is a need to call in a consultant who is a specialist in another field. These specialists are senior physicians who have trained and studied one subject for a long time, often acquiring advanced degrees. The burn patient might see any one or several of the following specialists.

The anesthesiologist. The entire burn team performs surgical procedures such as skin grafting and is customarily headed by the attending physician during the surgery. In this effort, the team is joined by the anesthesiologist, who makes critical decisions about the type and amount of anesthetic the patient should receive and monitors the patient's respiration, pulse, and blood pressure during surgery.

The cardiologist (heart specialist). For older people and for anyone with a history of heart disease or coronary disease, a major burn places great strain on the heart. The frequent need for surgical intervention to cover the burn wound, requiring general anesthesia, stresses the heart further. More rarely, infectious complications, which are a major threat to burn patients, can also affect the heart. For these reasons, the cardiologist is a frequent visitor to the burn unit who may be found in consultation with the burn team. The burn team calls upon the expertise of the cardiologist to help with the management of patients with cardiac problems.

The pulmonologist (lung specialist). Because smoke inhalation and other pulmonary complications of burns are very common, it is also natural that the lung specialist should be called upon frequently for help in treating patients in the burn unit. From time to time, pneumonia or other forms of lung infections set in. These infections can be life-threatening and difficult to clear with conventional techniques such as antibiotics.

In such instances, a procedure called a *bronchoscopy* is sometimes performed. During a bronchoscopy, the physician passes a very narrow, flexible tube inside the lung. With the sophisticated system of optics which is attached to the tube, the physician is able to see inside the lung and can then suction or clear out infected material. A bronchoscopy is usually performed by the lung specialist or a related specialist skilled in performing the procedure.

The psychiatrist or psychologist. Fully one-quarter of burn patients experience severe psychological or psychiatric disturbances. The severity of the disturbance varies from mild depression to delirium, which may include delusions and alterations in state of consciousness. In addition, many patients with burns have a previous underlying history of substance abuse—abuse of drugs or alcohol, or both. This problem, naturally, complicates the treatment of a stressful injury such as a burn. Psychiatrists (who have an M.D. degree and are licensed to prescribe drugs) and psychologists (who often have a Ph.D. degree and cannot prescribe drugs) are often called in to help the burn team with the treatment of patients who have problems with mental disturbances. These specialists are also available to care for patients who have persistent psychological problems after their physical recovery is accomplished and they have returned home from the hospital. (Psychological problems are discussed further in Chapter 5.)

The pediatrician. With small children and infants, there are pediatric needs in addition to the needs of the patient as burn victim. Pediatricians help the burn team with these problems. For example, a small child with a burn may develop a high fever not from the burn but from an illness or disease that any child might have, such as an infection of the middle ear. As a specialist in the care of children, the pediatrician is a helpful consultant to the burn team.

The nephrologist (kidney specialist). Kidney failure is common in burn patients and may be so severe that dialysis, or treatment with an artificial kidney machine, becomes necessary. The nephrologist is the specialist who consults with the burn team in setting up the schedule of dialysis. The dialysis machine is large and complex, and it performs a necessary function. Kidney failure due to burn injury is usually transient and temporary, and dialysis is usually required for only a few days or weeks.

The Nursing Team

Nurses provide much of the primary care of burn patients. They change dressings, administer injections, dispense medications, and do dozens of other things throughout the day and night to make the patient comfortable and promote his recovery. A nurse is a person who is knowledgeable about nursing procedures and medical science.

The nursing team is composed of professionals using their specific knowledge, training, experience, and background to help people overcome their burn injury and recover as quickly as possible to their fullest potential. Although the different members of the nursing team described in this section may sound vastly different from one another, they are all equally important, and they must work together as an integrated team to provide quality care for the burn patient.

Burn patients pose a challenge for the nursing team: they demand the best from the nurse physically, emotionally, and as human beings. Nurses who have been in burn care for a long time know that burn nurses are special people who are very proud of their accomplishments. But burn patients are always rewarding as they make progress in recovering. Burn nurses think of both their patients and themselves as very special people—which indeed they are.

The head nurse or nurse unit manager

As do most nursing units, the burn unit has a head nurse. The head nurse is usually a registered nurse who has a bachelor's degree, master's degree, or even a doctorate in nursing. She or he is usually practiced as a burn nurse. The job of head nurse is an administrative position; in fact, in many units the term *head nurse* is no longer used—other terms, such as *nursing manager* or *nurse unit manager,* may be used.

The head nurse is responsible, in part, for hiring new nurses and counseling the staff. One of the most important duties of the head nurse is gauging the number of nurses required to provide adequate care of patients on a day-to-day basis. In order to accomplish this, the head nurse must know the patients well.

The head nurse is also a financial manager, unless there is a separate business manager assigned by the hospital administration to the burn unit. The head nurse or a delegate is responsible for the ordering of nursing supplies such as bandages, dressings, burn cream, medications, and other items used in burn care. The head nurse reports administratively to a supervisor who in turn reports directly to the nursing administration of the hospital.

In addition to these administrative duties, the head nurse is responsible for the clinical nursing care of all patients on her unit, and she is expected to be familiar with the patients and their specific problems. Some head nurses focus only on the administrative responsibilities and seldom do "hands on" bedside nursing care. Others prefer to keep a hand in by doing bedside care from time to time. In many units, the head nurse may be required to function as an "emergency" backup and work as a regular floor nurse in cases of multiple admissions, acute unanticipated staff shortages, and other emergency situations.

Obviously, one talent that a modern head nurse must have is the ability to delegate portions of his responsibility to other senior members of his staff. The head nurse acts as a liaison between the medical staff and the nursing staff, and between the nursing staff and other parts of the hospital, from engineering to housekeeping.

The charge nurse

The first in line to assume responsibility from the head nurse is the charge nurse. The charge nurse is a registered nurse who at any point in time may be in charge of the unit. She or he reports directly to the head nurse. In some burn units a specific nurse is the permanent charge nurse for a certain shift: day shift, evening shift, or night shift. In other places, there is only a permanent day shift charge nurse. Then again, in some places, the "charge" rotates among different personnel at different times. In other units, depending on volume and traffic, there may not be a need for a charge nurse at all, if the head nurse can handle all charge duties.

The charge nurse may or may not have a bachelor's degree but generally has had several years of experience as a burn nurse. She is responsible for daily activities, including the provision of adequate supplies and medications. She also goes on rounds with the doctors (see below), gathers information on all patients, accepts admissions and transfers from other hospitals, ensures that the nursing staff is adequate to meet the needs of the patients, and makes patient assignments for the staff.

Assigning nurses to care for patients is probably the most important task of the charge nurse. He must make sure that the nurses can handle their assignments, obtaining assistance from other staff members when needed. The charge nurse himself usually has a patient assignment as well. Another important role is hour-by-hour problem solving with the staff. In the daily affairs of a burn unit, problems often arise with other departments in the hospital. It is up to the charge nurse to pursue and straighten out these problems whenever possible, since staff nurses (who have the major patient assignments) are often too busy to talk directly to members of other departments to attempt to solve problems. Like the head nurse, the charge nurse acts as a liaison between the doctors and the nurses. Both the head nurse and the charge nurse must have diplomatic talents to keep the unit running smoothly.

The unit nurse educator

The nurse educator is usually a registered nurse who has worked as a burn nurse for several years and has special skills in teaching.

This position is sometimes titled *nurse clinician, clinical nurse specialist,* or *education nurse*. These jobs may vary in detail, but they do not vary in substance. Teaching techniques also vary from unit to unit, depending on burn unit size, patient volume, and type of hospital (university teaching, community teaching, or general hospital). Regardless of these variables, the nurse educator's primary function is to provide staff education. The nurse educator helps establish and maintain a level of competency for new recruits and seasoned staff members and thereby plays a critical role in recruitment and retention of staff.

In some units, there is an extensive orientation period for new nurses. Orientation is the responsibility of the unit educator. Classes and formal lectures are given by a multidisciplinary teacher, and burn care courses are also taught. An incoming nurse is often engaged in orientation for several weeks or months before he or she is allowed independent patient responsibility. In other units, a "preceptor" system is used, where the unit educator assigns the new nurse to one of the veterans and the two work together until competence develops.

It is the responsibility of the unit educator to alert the nursing staff to advancements and new treatment in burn care and to supervise research in the use of new burn creams, medications, dressings, and other items that show promise of improving burn patient comfort and outcome. He or she helps the staff nurses keep their skills and knowledge current, through ongoing classes and demonstrations of new treatments and equipment. In this way, the staff nurses stay up to date on burn therapy. The unit educator may also function as a hands-on staff nurse and care for patients in the unit.

The staff nurse

The staff nurse is the backbone of the nursing staff. He or she is the nurse who is most frequently seen taking care of patients. Both patients and families have the closest relationship with the staff nurse, and they will turn to the staff nurse with their questions.

Staff nurses are registered nurses or licensed practical nurses working in the burn unit. They care for a patient from admission to discharge. They work in shifts, usually either 8 or 12 hours a day, and will often take care of the same patient day after day. The staff nurse therefore gets to know the patient very well and often gets to know the families well, too.

Because burn patients sometimes have a very long stay—up to several months—staff nurses tend to become attached to their patients. It is a most rewarding and wonderful experience to see a patient who has fought through a traumatic injury literally walk out of the burn unit and to know that you have had an impact on her recovery and her life. Of course, because of the need for the nurses to take time off, it is not possible or perhaps even desirable for all patients to have the *same* nurse for all of their care; nevertheless, individual knowledge of a patient is very important, and charge nurses and staff nurses attempt to assign the same staff members to a patient as often as possible.

It is a good idea for the family (or the patient, if the patient is well enough) to know at any point in time who "their" nurse is. Many patients, years after recovery, remember "their" nurse fondly and will make a special effort when returning to the hospital for therapy or outpatient visits to stop by the burn unit and show the nursing staff how well they're doing.

Other nursing personnel

Burn technicians, nursing aids, and others. In most burn care facilities, staff nurses are supplemented by a variety of trained individuals such as burn technicians and nursing aids who, although they are not licensed nurses, are very helpful in the daily care of the patient. The educational background of these individuals varies widely, but they all share one attribute: they have been educated and specially trained in burn care. Many of them remain in burn care throughout their career. Like staff nurses, they are given individual patients by the charge nurse. They can perform dressing changes and hydrotherapy (tubbing), help with critical patients, take vital signs, stock supplies, keep the unit neat and clean, and help the patients with daily care (baths, brushing teeth, washing hair, and feeding). They help nurses in the critical care areas by performing tasks such as mixing tube feedings and suctioning or clearing a patient's mouth. Designated duties may cover a wide array of procedures administered under the supervision of nurses. Their primary purpose is to assist with the nursing care of the burn patients.

The ward clerk. If there is any spot in a burn unit which could be compared to a strategic headquarters, it is undoubtedly the area occupied by the ward clerk or ward secretary. If you stand for five minutes in such an area and watch, you likely will feel as if you're in Times Square. The ward clerk's station is the telephone headquarters of the unit, often having four, five, or more extensions for communications. It is the ward clerk's job to answer the telephone and direct incoming inquiries to the person in the best position to answer that inquiry. The telephones might be ringing simultaneously with a call from the press inquiring about the latest method of burn therapy, from the police inquiring about an individual brought in after a suspicious fire, from a family member who has just heard that a loved one is in the hospital, and from a doctor needing an important question answered.

The ward clerk or secretary may also help keep supplies in the unit, file documents, keep the charts up to date, report laboratory results to the nurses, and gather admission information when a patient first comes into the unit. He or she acts as a link between the patient's family and the burn unit staff and informs families of the rules and visiting hours in the unit. On most burn services, it is also the ward clerk's duty to transcribe the doctor's orders onto the nurses' order sheet and thereby provide a vital link between the physicians and the nurses.

Other Medical Personnel

The physician's assistant. The physician's assistant is less knowledgeable than a physician and has trained differently than a nurse. Physician's assistants, who have completed two to four years of specialized training, must continually update their education and training and must practice under the supervision of a physician. A physician's assistant is licensed to perform various tasks, though the tasks a physician's assistant can be licensed to perform vary from state to state.

The nurse practitioner. The nurse practitioner is a registered nurse who has additional training and provides a middle level of care. Like the physician's assistant, the nurse practitioner can order tests and make recommendations for treatment, but the nurse practitioner does not have to be directly supervised by a physician.

The medical student. When the burn unit is affiliated with a university, it is possible for medical students to rotate through the unit, and the unit is frequently a favorite rotation for young students, who can learn a great deal by watching more experienced physicians manage the complex problems of burn patients. The student, in turn, is a valuable member of the team, often staying in the hospital at night to help the resident physicians.

Rounds

When a group of physicians and other health care professionals go "around" to see all the patients, it is said they are "on rounds." This team of professionals may have many seriously ill patients to see. Because of this the team often moves quickly, with the senior people at the head and the students at the tail, and may remind an observer of a comet.

Sometimes the group pauses outside a patient's door to talk in subdued tones, and then they look more like a football team in a huddle. The professionals who are "on rounds" confer with one another about each patient's care, discuss the results of recent diagnostic tests, and make decisions based on their observations and the test results.

Generally patients are not treated during rounds, because immediate treatment is not the purpose of rounds. Rather, rounds are designed primarily to provide information to the professionals and to help them plan the patient's treatment program together as a team. Patients and their families need not be afraid of the team on rounds, however, or feel that the members of the team don't want to answer questions. It may well be that the team does not have time to answer questions during rounds, but they can always make time to return to the patient's room when rounds are over.

One patient laughed out loud when the medical team arrived to visit "on rounds." She was embarrassed because she had laughed, though, and immediately apologized for thinking the team looked funny. It occurred to the members of the team that they may indeed have looked funny, shuffling around with all that pomp and ceremony.

Medical Procedures and Equipment

Sophisticated devices are used throughout the burn unit both to monitor and to treat patients. These machines are indispensable to the care of patients in the unit.

It is sometimes necessary for the physician to perform specific medical procedures when these machines are first put into use. Before performing any of these procedures which might be painful, the physician sedates the patient if the patient's condition permits this. The burn team never assumes that a patient who is comatose (in a coma) does not feel pain; therefore, all patients are given proper *anesthetic* (an agent that blocks the sensation of pain) or an *analgesic* (an agent that alleviates pain).

What follows is a description of the technology most commonly used in burn units and the procedures that accompany the use of this technology.

The monitor

The *monitor* (Figure 3.1) is an electronic box that is usually mounted on the wall close to the patient's bed, on a central power column, or on a stand. The monitor, as its name implies, monitors the patient. It does this by interpreting the several kinds of vital information it receives from tubes and wires leading from the patient's body to the monitor. Most monitors can decipher informa-

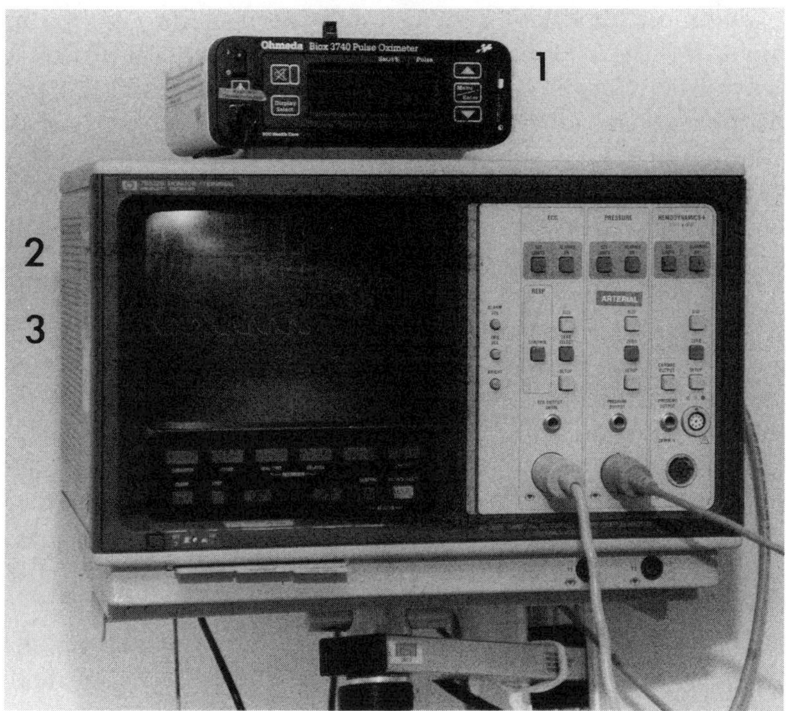

Figure 3.1. The monitor, showing (1) the pulse oximeter, which measures oxygen levels in the patient's blood; (2) the electrocardiogram; and (3) the blood pressure. Additional body systems can be measured by the monitor as required.

tion from four, five, or six inputs at the same time. The task of the monitor is to alert the burn team if the information it receives indicates that something about the patient's condition has changed significantly.

Sometimes the signals from room monitors are displayed at the nurses' station or another place to provide central monitoring. This way, the nurses can watch several patients' monitors at one time. The monitor may be connected to a memory computer, which can recall the monitoring from hours or days past, for comparison purposes. Some burn units also have a wall- or ceiling-mounted television camera that continuously sends an image of the patient directly to the nurses' station.

The most important kind of information monitored by the monitor is the information about a patient's heartbeat, which is provided by the EKG, or *electrocardiograph.* With an EKG, the patient has several adhesive pieces of plastic fixed to his body; wires attached to these pieces of plastic run out to the monitor to provide a continuous record of the variations in the electrical activity of the heart muscle. The electrical activity of the heart muscle can be detected through the skin, on the surface of the body.

The EKG produces a visual image, a wavelike pattern, on a screen resembling a television screen. As long as everything is going well, only this visual image is produced. When the monitor receives information from the EKG which indicates that the patient's heart muscle is showing abnormal activity, however, the monitor emits a warning sound, and the burn team comes running to the patient's room. It's not uncommon for a patient to dislodge a piece of plastic by moving around, and in these cases, the monitor has sounded a false alarm. Nevertheless, the sound of the monitor is always heeded by the burn team.

The monitor also keeps watch over the patient's blood pressure, since it is not practical for someone to stand at the bedside and constantly take a blood pressure reading the traditional way, with a cuff and stethoscope. To provide information to the monitor about blood pressure, physicians place a small plastic tube into one of the patient's arteries, in the wrist, foot, or groin. This is called the *arterial line,* or *A-line.* The tube is connected to an electronic device called a transducer, which converts the blood pressure into an electronic signal. Like the EKG, this signal produces a wavelike line on the monitor's screen.

Just as the arterial blood pressure can be monitored, so other pressures, in veins and in various parts of the heart, can be monitored, through tubes called *catheters.* The pressure measured by a catheter can be displayed on the monitor's screen as well. One kind of catheter, called the *Swan-Ganz catheter,* is frequently used to monitor critically ill people; this soft catheter has a balloon at the tip for measuring arterial pressure in the lung and provides information about the circulation that the other "lines" cannot.

The amount of oxygen in the patient's blood and the patient's rate of respiration are other body functions that can be monitored by the electronic device known as the monitor. The oxygen-measuring part of the monitor is called the *pulse oximeter*. Oxygen levels in the blood may be measured by attaching an oximeter to the patient's ear or finger or by directly measuring the oxygen content of arterial blood.

Oxygen levels in the blood are of particular significance in burn patients (this is more fully discussed in Chapter 1). An adequate oxygen concentration in blood is necessary to promote healing, to keep the heart working optimally, and to provide tissue cells with enough oxygen for adequate function.

Under normal conditions, the lungs translate air into an adequate concentration of oxygen for the blood through the process of respiration. Most people who are not seriously ill can get adequate oxygen from the air and need no supplemental oxygen supply. But most burn patients, at least in the early stages of their recovery, need some form of supplementation; this is most easily provided with a face mask or nasal prongs attached to the oxygen source in the wall. If the patient's lungs are so seriously injured that this amount of oxygen cannot be translated by the lungs into an adequate concentration for the blood, then the patient must be supported by a respirator, as discussed below.

The respirator

The *respirator* (Figure 3.2), also called the ventilator (or "vent"), helps a person breathe. There are many reasons why a person with serious burns cannot breathe well. Inhaled smoke may cause swelling that obstructs the patient's airway, or the patient may have pneumonia. Sometimes there is fluid in the lungs from the burn (this is common, particularly after smoke inhalation). In the event that the person cannot breathe properly, two steps must be taken to prevent suffocation. First, a tube called an *endotracheal tube* (or ET tube) is placed through either the mouth or the nose down the breathing pipe (or trachea), and then the ET tube is hooked up to a respirator, which is literally a breathing machine in that it breathes for the patient by pushing humidified oxygen and air into the patient's lungs in a cycle imitating the person's normal breathing cycle.

Having a tube down your throat is uncomfortable, and patients don't like it. Nor do they like having a machine breathing for them. But it is dangerous when a patient fights the respirator, and

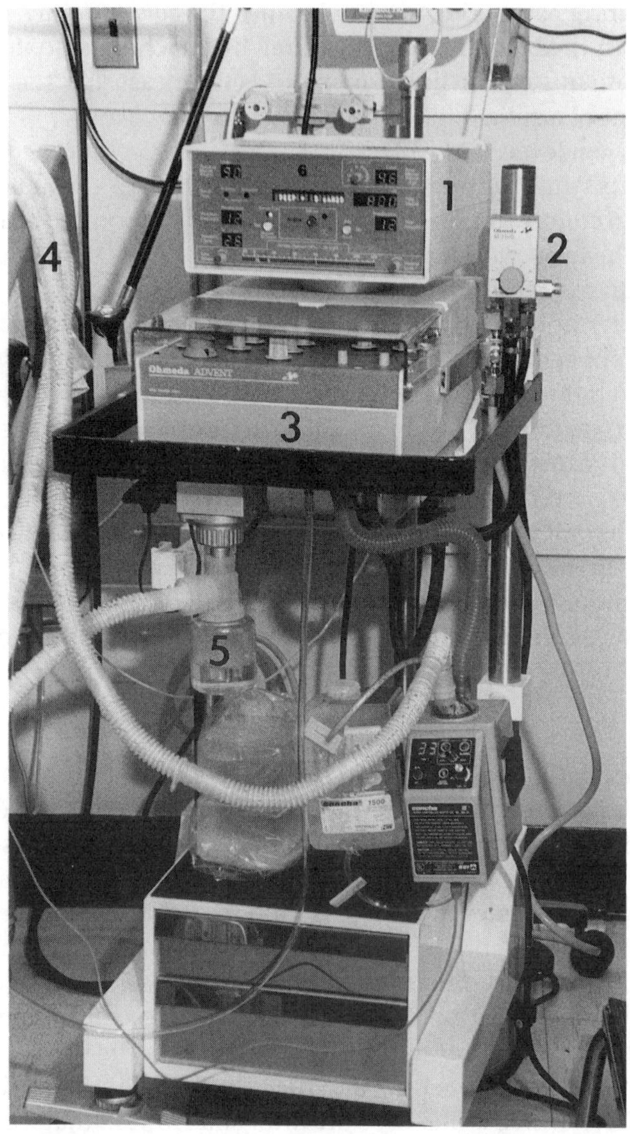

Figure 3.2. The respirator. (1) Numbers display the patient's respiratory rate, volume of air being breathed by the machine for the patient, and other details. (2) Adjustment can be made for the percentage of oxygen being delivered to the patient; this is called the "FIO tube." (3) The knobs for adjusting the patient's respiratory rate, volume of air, and so on. (4) The air tube leading to and from the patient. (5) The humidifier provides inspired air.

any struggle against this machine must be stopped: the machine is stronger than the patient, and it can hurt the patient who fights against it. Also, sometimes patients pull out the ET tube.

In order to protect the patient against harm, and in order to allow the respirator to do its job, all patients in the burn unit who are on respirators are sedated so they will tolerate the situation. Some people are so strong or so agitated that they cannot be sedated, and in that case they are paralyzed with drugs (usually pancuronium or Pavulon). Paralyzing drugs must be administered every few hours in order to sustain the paralysis, since this is the only way to protect these patients. Physical restraints are not sufficient to prevent people from fighting the ventilator.

After a number of days, usually between the 10th day and the 20th day on the respirator, the ET tube can become very irritating to the nose or mouth. When this happens, a *tracheostomy* is performed, usually under local anesthetic. A tracheostomy is a surgical opening in the windpipe through which a tracheostomy tube—a shorter version of the ET tube—is passed. This arrangement is usually more comfortable for the patient and allows the medical staff to care for the tube with a minimal amount of discomfort for the patient.

Sometimes health care professionals use an "insider's" vocabulary when they speak with each other. When a health care professional says "Beth, watch 84 while I go on break. He's pavulonized on the vent," she means "Beth, watch Mr. Jones in room 84 for a while. He is paralyzed and on a respirator." To an observer, this way of talking may appear somewhat insensitive, but this "shorthand" way of communicating allows health care professionals to communicate quickly and efficiently with their colleagues, and this kind of communication is often crucially important, especially under emergency circumstances.

Lines and tubes

Just as sailors call their ropes *sheets*, physicians call their small tubes *lines* (though a *large* tube is called a tube). Tubes are usually made of plastic and are usually clear; they may be flexible or rigid. Some examples of tubes are the endotracheal tube and the arterial blood pressure tube, or A-line, discussed above. Burn patients may have other tubes in their body as well.

Lines that are placed into the patient's veins are called *intravenous lines* (or IVs). These are the lines most commonly used in medical care. IVs can supply tissue-bathing fluids, nutrients, antibiotics, analgesics, and other medications, as well as blood, directly to the patient's circulatory system. Often it is necessary to administer solutions that are not compatible with each other (for example, blood and nutrition fluid cannot be given to the patient through the same IV line). For this reason, several IV lines—sometimes as many as four separate lines—may have to be placed in the patient.

A tube placed in the patient's bladder is called a urinary catheter or a *Foley catheter*. Using the natural force of gravity, this catheter drains urine from the bladder. The urine is stored in a urine bag, so the patient's output of urine can be measured. The Foley sometimes causes discomfort when it is first inserted, but most people adjust to it quickly. Removal of a patient's Foley catheter is a clear sign of improvement.

A tube inserted through the nose or mouth into the stomach is called a *nasogastric tube* (or NG tube). This tube serves a dual function: soon after the burn injury, when the stomach is not functioning, the nasogastric tube is used to suction the stomach contents out of the stomach. This keeps the stomach empty and prevents the patient from vomiting or aspirating stomach contents into his lungs, which can cause pneumonia. After the patient's stomach resumes its normal function, the nasogastric tube can be used to feed the patient. A smaller tube can often be used for this purpose. Even after the patient has recovered sufficiently to be able to eat on her own, this tube may be left in for supplemental feeding, because most people cannot eat enough to satisfy the enormous caloric requirements of burn patients.

A tube in the patient's intestine, called a *jejunostomy tube* or gastrostomy tube, makes long-term feeding possible and is often used when the patient's ability to swallow has been affected by his injury. A pump, gravity, or intermittent syringefuls can be used to deliver nutrients to the patient through the gastrostomy tube. These nutrients are individually prescribed for the needs of the specific patient, and their delivery is carefully monitored by the medical staff. These tubes may be inserted surgically.

For the patient and the family, one of the most important things to remember about tubes is that they are not permanent: as the patient improves and no longer needs to be as closely monitored or to receive nutrients through a tube, for example, tubes are removed. Some tubes, such as the endotracheal tube, must be removed over several days or weeks (this process is called "weaning"), and removing a tracheostomy takes even longer, as the patient gradually relearns to breathe on his own.

Other technology

Figure 3.3 depicts the setting of a modern intensive care room. In addition to the respirator (located to the left of the patient's bed), the room contains a heat shield; wall sockets providing suction, oxygen, and air; an automatic intravenous infusion pump; and a urine bag (just visible near the bottom of the bed rail). The room's monitor is to the right of the patient's bed, almost out of the picture.

The body's ability to retain heat is compromised in burn patients, so it is necessary to keep them warm mechanically, through heat radiated by a *heat shield*. Most people who suffer a severe burn injury remain under a heat shield until they are nearly completely healed.

Through a face mask or a tube, a patient receives oxygen and air that is delivered throughout the hospital through a system whose openings in the patient's room are the *wall sockets*. One wall socket delivers oxygen and another delivers air to the patient. In addition, two other sockets provide suction force, which can be used by medical personnel to clear mucus and other body fluids from the patient's throat and lungs and to suction the stomach and other body cavities.

The *automatic intravenous infusion pump* pumps fluids through the intravenous lines into the patient's circulatory system. Each drug fluid requires a separate pump, so it is not unusual for there to be as many as six or seven pumps in a patient's room. The intravenous infusion pumps are mounted on intravenous poles, which may be moved about the room if necessary.

As noted above, the urine bag is the receptacle into which the Foley catheter empties. The urine collected in that bag is mea-

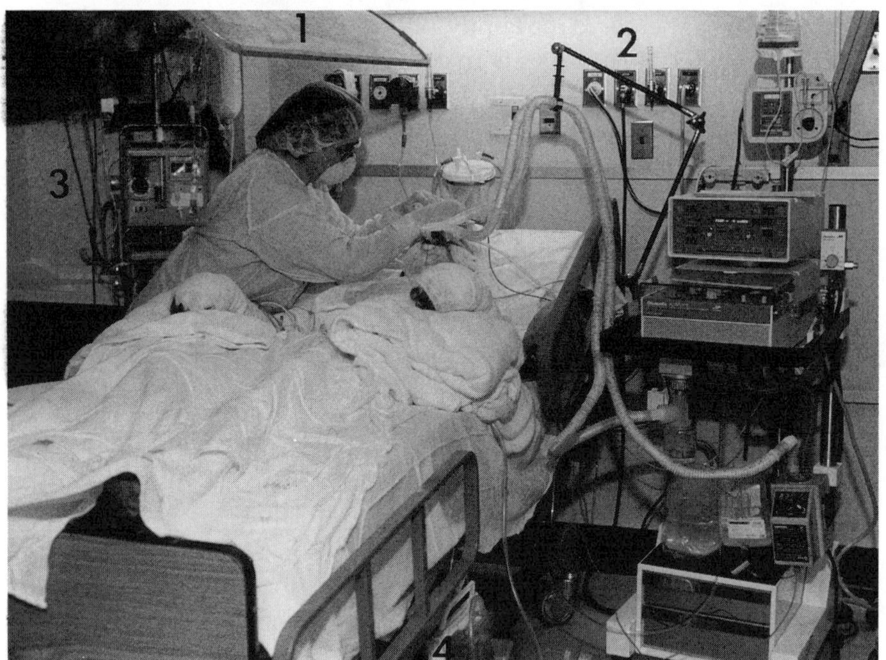

Figure 3.3. The setting of a modern intensive care room. (1) The heat shield maintains the patient's body temperature. (2) Wall sockets provide oxygen, air, and suction. (3) The automatic intravenous infusion pump; one of these is required for each fluid being administered, so it is not unusual for patients to have as many as six or seven of these machines mounted on various IV poles. (4) The urine bag is used for measuring the patient's hourly output of urine.

sured, usually on an hourly basis. Measurement of the patient's output of urine allows the burn team to determine whether the internal organs, especially the kidneys, are functioning properly, and to monitor the patient's state of hydration.

Part II

The Road to Recovery

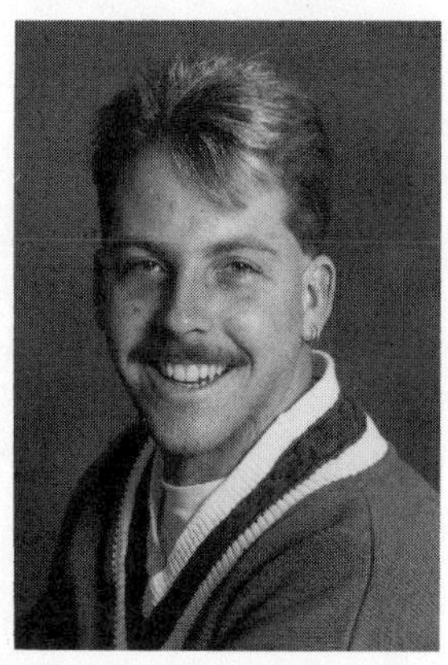

While I was at work on April 7, 1986, something happened that changed the course of my life. I was electrocuted and burned over 45 percent of my body. I'm going to share with you the many stages I went through and the many feelings I felt. In my opinion, everybody deals with things in their own way. I was eventually able to deal with my accident, but the stages and phases a burn patient goes through in the beginning are sketchy, because the mind has a way of blocking out bad things.

First of all, I can remember being taken by an ambulance to St. Agnes Hospital. I was intubated there, then transferred to the Baltimore Regional Burn Center. When I first woke up at the Burn Center, I remembered everything that happened for the first few days. As the days passed, though, I started forgetting the details of the accident. I could not even remember what happened. My head hurt very badly. It felt like someone had dropped something very heavy on my head. Finally, I started to remember where I was and why I was in the hospital. I did not want to be there.

The doctors talked to my parents and to me. They explained the gravity of the situation and what my chances were for recovery. The doctors also told them what to expect over this long ordeal. My parents were told that I would fade in and out from the pain and painkillers and that I could become disoriented. Early on, I was overtaken with severe depression. Ultimately, it lasted my entire two-month hospital stay. The depression was much more severe in the beginning and then less severe toward the end of my stay.

While I was in the hospital, I had terrible dreams that people were hurting me. After a while, the nightmares subsided. I would fall asleep for a few minutes, wake up, and think it was the next day. Hours and days would just run together. To help me keep track of time, my father took big sheets of paper and wrote the days of the week on them. He did this so I could be clear in my mind what day it was when I awoke.

An especially unpleasant phase was when I thought I was losing my mind. I couldn't believe that I, a 19-year-old boy, was having these strange feelings of depression and helplessness. My hands were so badly burned that I could not move, eat, drink, or even go to the bathroom by myself. With all these things, I asked to see a psychiatrist. He came to see me, and he kept coming for almost a month. He really helped me deal with some of my problems.

Another phase was when I needed desperately to let my family know how much I love them. I had such an urgency to tell them I loved them so very much. Before my accident, I was a 19-year-old tough guy who wouldn't tell anybody that I loved them. Since I felt that I might die, I wanted them to know how much I really did dearly love and appreciate them. I asked my mom to call my sister, who was in Georgia, to tell her for me just how much I loved her. I also had a lot of anxieties about never having a pretty girlfriend, and I knew that I would never again go to Ocean City and lay on the beach. I would never be able to let anybody see me without my shirt because of my scars.

I was just so afraid of everything around me. The doctors would say one thing, and I would think they had said something else. This upset me to the point of near-hysteria. The nurse would want to know what I was so upset about, and I would tell her and she would laugh because she couldn't believe the craziness that I had thought up. Everything for me was confusing.

One of the hardest things to do while lying in bed in pain is to eat a hearty meal. Eating is essential for the healing process of a burn patient, but I would take one or two bites of food and be stuffed. The lack of appetite makes it hard to eat, even though you must eat to heal. I had to learn to eat with a fork or spoon that was fastened to a bracelet on my wrist. It was frustrating at first, but once I got the hang of it, I could feed myself. Nicely, I regained a little independence, and I knew I was on the road to recovery.

Today, five years later, I live in Ocean City with my beautiful girlfriend. I lead a very happy and productive life thanks to the help and support of family and friends at the Baltimore Regional Burn Center.

Bob Campbell

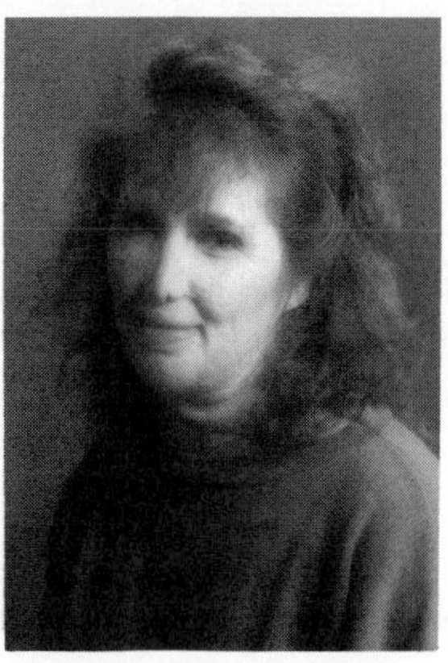

It was Easter Sunday and the nurses kept saying "You're in Shock-Trauma" as they were washing my hair. Well my scalp, really. All my long, blond hair had been burned or shaved off, and I was sitting in a chair for the first time. Everyone seemed to know me, but I recognized no one. I could not talk because I had a tracheostomy. I couldn't move my hands because they were so badly contracted with burns. I couldn't move much of anything, as my body had atrophied from being in a special Clinitron bed and immobile for six weeks; I had been in a coma.

I knew I was lucky to be alive and I felt grateful—ecstatic, even. My mother and brother came to see me that day. For two weeks my prognosis for survival had remained slim. Then, as I strengthened, the doctors told them that I might never see or hear again. They weren't sure if I would ever function outside a nursing home. They couldn't gauge the extent of the trauma damage until I awoke. I found out that I had been smoking in bed, and later I found out that I had been drinking also, even though I was a recovering alcoholic.

I had third-degree burns on 30 percent of my body. My whole face and neck were deeply burned. I had lost my nose. Both my hands were third degree, but I hadn't lost any fingers. My lower abdomen and left thigh were burned down to the muscle, so that it looked like chunks of me were missing. My right arm and right leg were also burned. I had no memory of the house fire or of the few preceding days. My children had been at my mother's house.

Being in the critical care unit was very disorienting and frightening. I have three sons and a daughter who were ages 6 through 15 then, and I missed them. I had imagined I would bounce from the bed now and walk down the hall, but it was painful to take steps into a chair 3 feet away. I began to hate my therapists. Every exercise hurt, and the braces on my neck and hands were uncomfortable. When the therapist left, I would beg the nurses to let me take them off. The nurses said that the doctors had ordered them, so I started to resent most of the doctors and the nurses then, too. I would do anything they said because I thought this would get me home sooner. When I got home, everything would be all right.

Before I could go home, my children had to come to the hospital to see if they could accept my appearance. They were wonderful, but they were nervous, and so was I. We moved into my mother's split-level house. I could barely get up the steps to the living room. Looking in the mirror at the hospital, I had anticipated seeing a burned face and a ravaged body. The last time I had glimpsed myself in the mirror at home, I had been attractive and vibrant. It just couldn't be me, I thought, but I knew it was because I felt awful. All I wanted to do was curl up in a ball and not have anyone touch me, because everything was sore and the donor sites and grafts felt strange. They hurt and felt separate at the same time.

Within a month, I was back in the hospital for the start of my reconstructive surgery. When I was home, I went to the hospital three times a week to see the doctors and for physical or occupational therapy. In and out of the hospitals was my life for a full year.

In the hospital everyone measured my progress from the day I entered, so by those standards I was only improving. At home, my family and I could only think how I used to be. At home there were pictures of me before the fire. In the living room sat the piano that I had played and the crocheted afghans I had made. In the yard was my garden I could not work and the car I could no longer drive.

At first I got a lot of cards, and a few phone calls, but they dwindled off. My best friend came over to the house but never returned. Another friend, my manager at work, promised to visit but never did. My world was changing. Another friend of mine visited, but he kept coming back. My plastic surgeon showed me that the people who were now taking care of me were willing to offer friendship and emotional support also.

Before the fire, I was a full-time bartender, so my free time was limited. I began to think that all this time now was a gift. I started making lists. I made a list of all the books I had always wanted to read and the places I hoped to visit. I started thinking of little things that I wanted. I wanted to smell good, not like hospital ointments, so I bought some great perfume. I started making an afghan as hand therapy. I made a list of performers I wanted to see in concert and the songs I wanted to play on the piano. I started practicing the piano again as therapy. My friend and I would plan trips in the future "after my operations, when it was all over," as I would say to myself. When I looked good again, I could enjoy these things.

And my life got a little better. But my operations were going on and on. I had many graft rejections and infections. My new nose looked good, but it was clear I would never be a conventional beauty again. When I went out in public, people noticed me. Some stared.

My long lists were not adequate coping mechanisms. They were just distractions and escapes. I realized that I didn't like myself at all anymore. I was afraid that no man could love me ever again. I couldn't imagine how anyone would hire me for a job. I was watching my children's lives like a spectator.

At night, I would wake from nightmares trembling and sweating, trying desperately to erase those visions. When the pounding of my heart and the throbbing in my eardrums slowed, I would slip on headphones, hoping music would calm me. I would rock back to sleep and dream, afraid to stay awake and think about life. I felt completely alone. Finally, 18 months after the fire, I drank again. I had given up. I became so ill that my stomach started bleeding, and I landed in another hospital for a month. I had risked the few precious things that I still had, my children's love and respect, my doctors' and friends' trust, and my life.

From that low point, I slowly improved. A year later, I took my first surgical break. The art and artifacts of the Smithsonian Institution in Washington, D.C., had brought me comfort and inspiration. In the summer of 1988, I started working there in a volunteer position. I took the train from Baltimore to Washington, and it was the first time since the fire that I had been on my own in public. It was scary but also thrilling to be independent again. I became very aware of my differences. I was still wearing the neck brace then and going to Francis Scott Key for my occupational therapy. The occupational therapists there told me of a burn survivor's support group that met weekly in the hospital.

One day, I saw my old friend and manager, and I was ashamed of the way I looked and angry still over her rejection. I knew I needed to talk about it. My family, in efforts to protect me, had staunchly denied that society was treating me differently now, but I knew better. At first, when I went to group, I mainly listened. I didn't know anyone there, but I recognized their stories. These stories of pain and long struggles interspersed with well-earned laughter were relief to me. After all, they were very familiar.

One day in group, I started talking about myself. I said, "Why can't my life be better than before?" A wise member asked, "What's stopping you?" I realized that in many ways I was preventing myself from enjoying life. I learned that when you leave the hospital and do the work it takes to get better, you are no longer a victim. You become a burn survivor. I finally admitted that that day in February 1986 had altered my life forever. I knew that I could never get that pretty, carefree, young woman back, but I had grown fond of the woman in her place. I know there are people in society who will never feel comfortable around me, and I don't let them control my life.

My two oldest boys are in college now. My only daughter is a bright, athletic high school student. My youngest son in middle school is just as active, and I am a full participant in their lives. I am still working at the Smithsonian, but as a paid employee now. I taught myself how to quilt, and I am now entering national competitions.

I've had over 30 operations. After two years, they became operations of choice more than necessity. My life is very different, but it is a good life. I am much stronger emotionally, if a bit sadder and wiser. My life is so busy now that my lists are full of things I have to do. I'm squeezing in the wishes from previous lists. When I leave my home, I do not worry about other people's reactions to me.

I don't have any specific physical limitations, though I tire more easily. I avoid too much exposure to the sun, but I like to feel its warmth on my face. A lot of my tactile sensation has returned. My scars are no longer red and raised. I attribute this to the Jobst garments, and the braces those hated therapists made me wear. Some of those therapists are my closest friends.

Rather than one day at a time, some days I felt I could only make it through one minute. Now I savor my moments. They are the times I'm sure of, and I want every one that is left for me.

Annie Kuebler

Chapter 4

Physical Rehabilitation

Most children and adults who have survived a burn injury are able to participate in the same activities at home and in the community which they took part in prior to their injury. This would include simple tasks such as dressing and bathing, as well as more complex tasks like cooking meals, cleaning house, and driving. Survivors of all ages benefit from recreational activities that can be done individually (swimming and needlework, for example) or with a group (softball, scouting). In addition, the adult survivor needs to return to the working world and the child or adolescent to school.

Through physical rehabilitation, the burn patient regains the skills necessary to accomplish these tasks easily and efficiently. The process of regaining joint motion, muscle strength, coordination, endurance, and other skills through physical therapy (PT) begins soon after admission to the burn unit and can continue for many months following discharge. The rehabilitation team is led by physical and occupational therapists, but the patient and the family must participate in order for the rehabilitation to be successful. The work of physical rehabilitation is hard, and it is often painful and emotionally tiring, but the long-term results make a significant difference in the life of the burn survivor.

The staff members who design the patient's PT program and then instruct and guide the patient through physical rehabilitation are the *physical therapist* and the *occupational therapist.* The physical therapist has earned either a four-year bachelor's degree or a six-year master's degree and has completed a clinical internship. The physical therapist's role in burn care is to return the burn survivor to independent functioning in all aspects of her life. This is accomplished through evaluation and treatment planning, promotion of wound healing, therapeutic exercise, mobility activities, and control of hypertrophic scarring. In addition, the physical therapist uses hot packs, ultrasound, and electrical stimulation to relieve the patient's pain and *edema*, or swelling.

The occupational therapist's role in burn care is to return the patient to the highest level of independent functioning possible. The patient's physical limitations and psychological condition are assessed and addressed by the occupational therapist. Like the physical therapist, the occupational therapist may have either a bachelor of science degree or a master's degree in occupational therapy. Occupational therapists obtain national certification through examination, and they must be licensed in the state in which they practice.

The Evaluation

A comprehensive evaluation of the patient is the first step in physical rehabilitation. The physical and occupational therapists complete the evaluation as soon as possible after the patient is admitted to the burn unit. The first portion of the evaluation involves obtaining general information (name, age), burn injury information (when and how the injury occurred), a medical history, and information about the patient's physical status before the burn (for example, did a 1-year-old walk by himself? Did an 80-year-old use a walker?). Family members often help the therapist by describing what the patient could and could not do before the burn injury. This step allows realistic expectations to be established.

Next, the therapist will assess the patient's alertness, ability to follow directions, and response to pain. The burn wound is inspected, and its depth (first, second, or third degree) and location are noted. Deeper burns—burns that require skin grafting—and burns that cross one or more joints can cause difficulties during rehabilitation.

The therapist also assesses the range of motion in all the patient's body joints, including the neck and trunk. *Range of motion* is the distance through which a joint can move. If motion is limited, the range of motion is measured with an instrument called a *goniometer*, which records the motion in numerical degrees (a normal elbow, for example, would range from 0 degrees when fully extended to approximately 135 degrees when fully flexed). Strength of individual muscle groups is tested if the patient is able to move actively.

Sensation is assessed next. The therapist notes decreased or absent sensation in both the burn wound and other, nonburned body areas. The patient's ability to move in bed by rolling and sitting up, and to use his or her hands for activities such as eating, is also analyzed. Finally, if the patient is able to be out of bed, his ability to walk is assessed.

When the evaluation is completed, the therapist will use the data obtained to establish short- and long-term treatment goals and will construct a daily treatment plan designed to help the patient reach those goals. After the initial evaluation, the burn patient will be reevaluated over the course of rehabilitation. Goals and treatment plans will be modified as the patient makes progress or suffers setbacks.

Positioning to Prevent Loss of Motion

A major concern of physical rehabilitation is preventing the loss of joint motion in a person who has sustained a burn injury. The inability to move a joint fully because of tightness of the surrounding tissue is called *contracture*. In burn patients, contracture occurs for two reasons. First, because the burned areas are painful, the patient assumes a position that lessens the pain and will remain in that position because it is more comfortable. If a joint is not moved, it will become tight, and eventually the person will not be able to move the joint at all. Second, as the burn heals, scar tissue sometimes develops. This tissue is not pliable and will pull tightly across the joints. Contractures can be prevented by range-of-motion exercises and proper positioning of the involved joints (Table 4.1).

The technique used most frequently for positioning is splinting. Many patients need splints soon after admission; others may not need a splint until later, when they become less mobile due to pain and skin tightness. If a skin graft is required across a joint, a splint will be fabricated in the operating room to immobilize the extremity properly and to protect the new graft. A splint is formed from a sheet of polymer and plastic which becomes malleable when heated. It is shaped to fit over the affected joint (Figure 4.1).

Table 4.1. Proper Positioning of Burned Joint Areas

Neck	Extended
Shoulder	Arms held out at shoulder height or above
Elbow	Extended
Wrist	Extended
Hand	
Index, middle, ring, little fingers	If burn on palm, all joints extended; if burn on top of hand, proximal joint bent, distal joints extended
Thumb	Out to side of hand
Hip	Extended and not turned in or out
Knee	Extended
Ankle	At 90° angle to leg, not turned in or out

Some patients benefit from wearing a commercially made splint that allows positioning in a range of joint motion. With these splints, the position of the joint can be frequently adjusted.

A splint should fit well and be fairly comfortable to wear. Some splints are worn continuously, and others are worn for specific periods during the day or night. The therapist will instruct the patient and family in caring for the splint and will give them a schedule for its use. The therapist will also answer any questions the patient or family may have.

Other devices, including pillows, rolled towels, and foam wedges, can be used to achieve proper positioning. Commercial devices are sometimes used to achieve the best positioning. Padded metal troughs that attach to the bed to achieve proper shoulder positioning are required by patients who have burns across their shoulders and are spending most of their time in an air bed (Figure 4.2).

The arms and legs may be elevated above heart level to decrease swelling, which is most common during the first few days of treatment. Patients may require elevation at other times, too, particularly after skin graft surgery.

As the patient begins to move more actively on her own, the need for splinting decreases. However, patients may need to continue to wear splints during the outpatient phase of their rehabilitation to prevent contractures due to scarring.

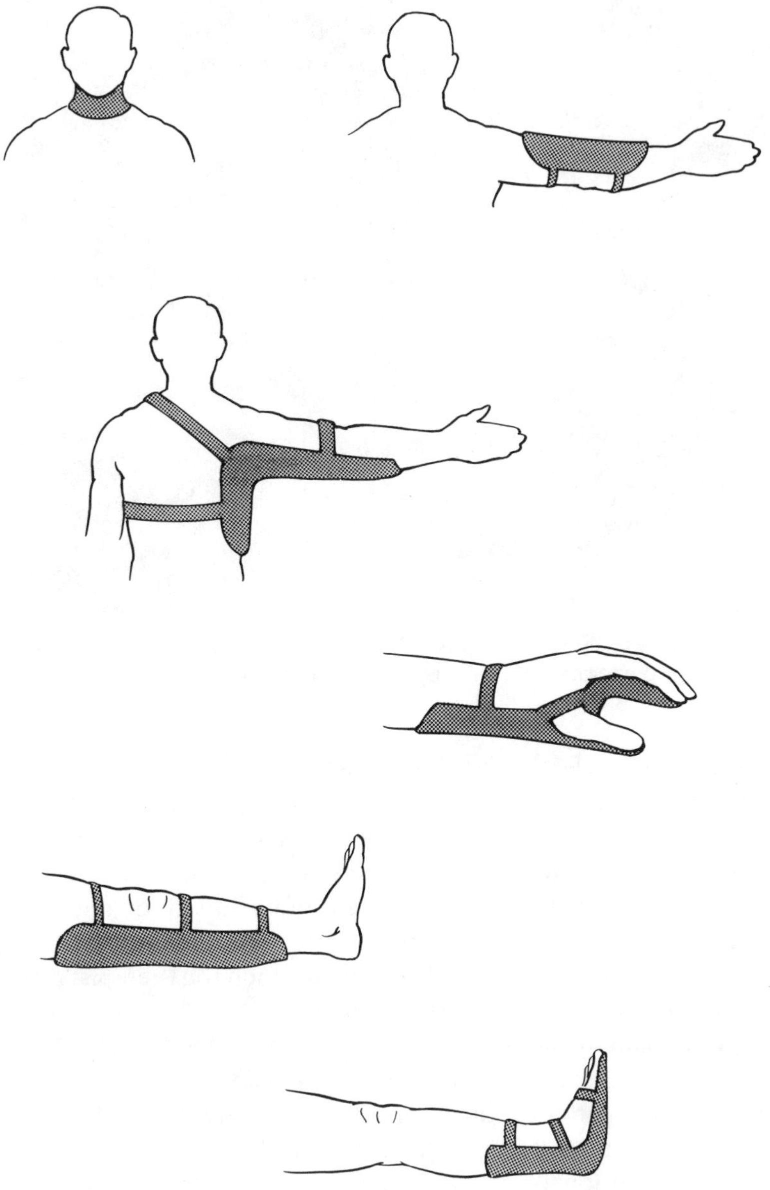

Figure 4.1. Splints such as these are used across joints to provide proper positioning and prevent the formation of contractures.

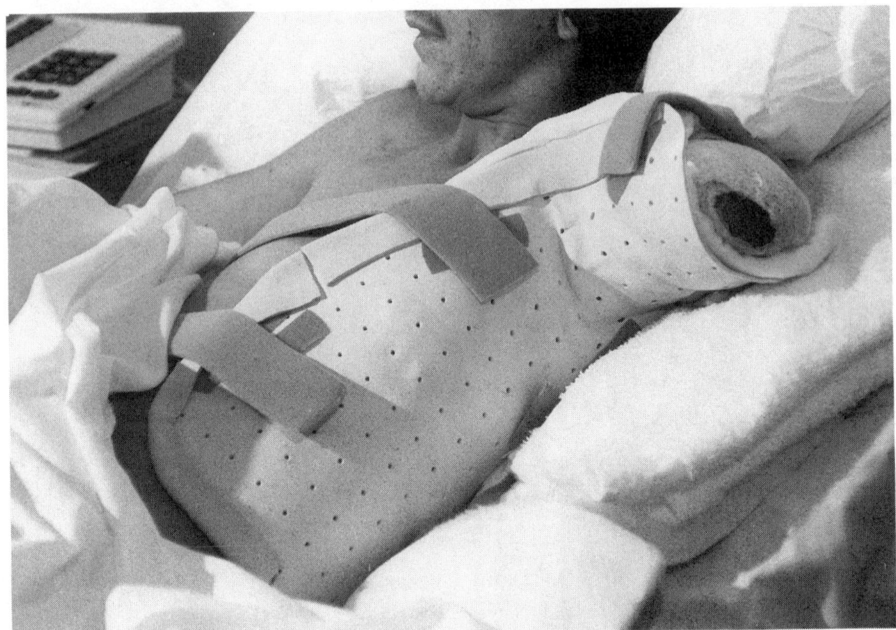

Figure 4.2. Positioning the limbs in a comfortable "position of function" is important preparation for the beginning of exercises.

Exercising to Regain Motion

The therapist begins working with the burn patient on an exercise program to restore active movement as soon as possible after the patient is admitted. Three basic exercise techniques are employed: (1) *active motion,* in which the patient moves on his own, without help; (2) *active assisted motion,* in which the therapist helps the patient move; and (3) *passive motion,* in which the therapist moves the patient without the patient's help.

Some patients are initially unable to move on their own, and the therapist needs to use the passive motion technique with them. As the patient's condition improves, active assisted and gentle active exercises are incorporated into the exercise program.

Active motion is the preferred exercise technique, since this technique not only moves the joints but helps to improve muscle strength. Although the exercise program will stress moving the body areas that were burned, unburned areas must also be exercised to prevent loss of motion and strength.

Exercise can be very painful. The therapist will work with the physician, psychologist, and other members of the burn unit staff to develop a program to help control pain during exercise sessions. Medication, relaxation, and imagery are frequently used to achieve relief from pain. Some patients prefer to exercise the most painful areas at the beginning of the therapy session, and some prefer to save those exercises for the end of the session. Bulky dressings may limit full motion, and sometimes exercises are done during tubbing, when the dressings are off. The tub has the added advantage of the buoyancy of water, which assists the patient's movement during exercise.

The exercise program needs to be performed at least once daily; ideally the patient gets together with the physical and occupational therapists twice daily for exercise sessions. The program may be interrupted if the patient's medical status is too critical to allow exercise, or following surgery, when the grafted area is immobilized for three to five days to help promote graft take.

As the burn wound heals, the exercise program stresses stretching of the skin and underlying structures in a slow, sustained manner. Areas of the face (especially surrounding the eyes and mouth), neck, and trunk need to be stretched, as do the extremities. Skin tightness caused by the scarring process can occur rapidly (see Chapter 1), can affect the underlying muscle, tendons, ligaments, and joints, and can continue until the scar is fully matured. The tightness and limited mobility may be relieved after exercise, only to return after a few hours. This regression can become a source of considerable frustration for the burn patient, who needs to be reassured and encouraged by the staff and by family members.

Staff members try to involve the patient in the development of exercise goals, because a burn survivor who is actively involved may be more motivated to do the hard work necessary to achieve these goals (Figure 4.3). Achieving a specific personal goal may be all that is needed to increase the patient's willingness to persevere with the exercise program.

A variety of devices and equipment may be employed in the exercise portion of the physical rehabilitation program. In fact, the number and type of devices and equipment are limited only by availability and the therapist's imagination. Simple devices include overhead pulleys, sandbag and barbell weights, elastic exer-

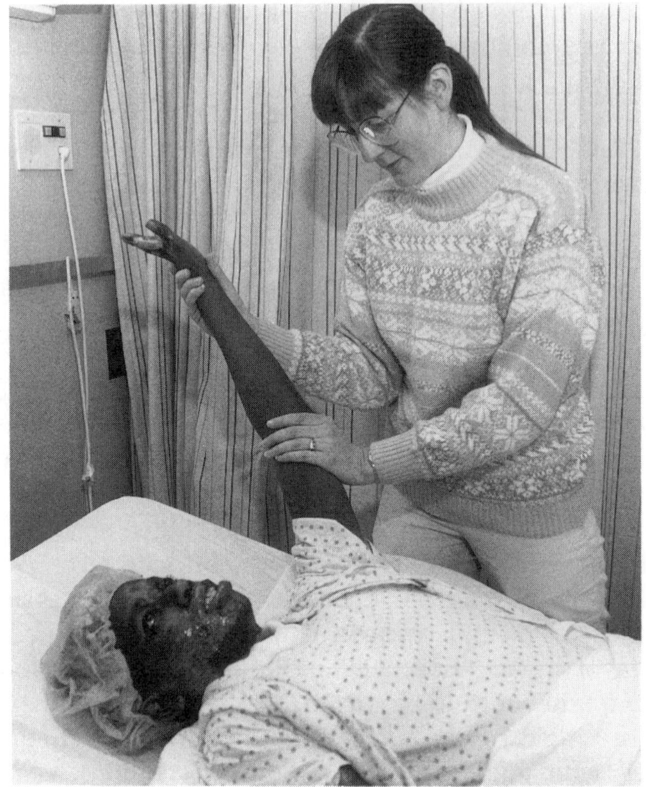

Figure 4.3. Careful early exercising under supervision speeds recovery.

cise bands or tubing, and hand grippers. More complex equipment includes bicycles, treadmills, upper- and lower-body ergometers, isokinetic machines (like those used by professional athletes), and work or activity simulation devices. In some parts of the world, therapeutic spring baths and even pressure water therapy are used to increase range of motion.

Mobility and Activities of Daily Living to Regain Function

Early mobility helps the patient physically and psychologically. Mobility includes rolling over in bed, sitting up in bed, moving from the bed to a stretcher, and sitting in a chair. Often mobility is a progression from simple to more complex activities, starting in bed and continuing until the patient can again move freely in the environment. When the patient is medically stable, he should be out of bed as much as possible. Even a patient who still has multiple IV lines, has a tracheostomy, is covered with bandages and splints, and has burns that have not yet healed may be out of bed.

One might think that resting in bed would be the best way to conserve energy and heal wounds, but that is not the case: lying in bed day after day produces serious side effects. Prolonged bed rest has a substantial negative impact on all the major systems of the body. Bed rest decreases lung volume or "vital capacity," for example, and this can lead to pneumonia.

Prolonged bed rest can affect the cardiovascular system as well as the respiratory system, in that it can cause a decrease in blood volume and a decrease in the number of red blood cells. This results in a decrease in the amount of oxygen available to the body and may interfere with the healing of wounds. Since the patient is lying down, gravity can't assist the heart's pumping action. Thus the heart must work harder. Also, blood can pool in veins, leading to blood clots that may contribute to infection or stroke. A rapid drop in blood pressure and fainting may occur when the patient who has been lying in bed begins sitting in a chair or standing. This is called *orthostatic hypotension.*

The musculoskeletal system can also be adversely affected by bed rest. Muscles can weaken by about 20 percent during one week of inactivity in bed. The muscles actually decrease in size, or atrophy. Motor strength is also affected. Risk of loss of bone density (*osteoporosis*) and accumulation of excess bone across joints (*heterotopic ossification*) or in muscle (*myositis ossificans*) increases as well. This new bone can cause pain and severely limit motion, and it may eventually have to be removed surgically.

Lying in one position too long can cause pressure sores to develop in the skin over bony prominences in both burned and unburned areas. Prolonged bed rest can also result in decreased appetite and constipation due to slowing of the bowel.

Besides physical complications, bed rest can lead to psychological problems. Boredom may be a result of being inactive and staying in the same room all the time. Decreased mobility results in increased dependency and loss of control, which can in themselves lead to depression. The patient who must be on bed rest may have great anxiety when attempting to regain mobility. She may be afraid of failure, pain, or falling or sustaining another injury. The therapist can ease the patient through these fears and show her how she can safely regain mobility.

The therapist will work hard to get the patient to help himself. From the time of admission the patient is encouraged to assist in rolling in bed, sitting up, lifting his upper body (often using a bed trapeze), and lifting his lower body. The patient will be taught how to help the staff in moving her from bed to stretcher to go to the tub or shower and how to change positions in the tub.

As soon as possible the patient will sit out of bed in a chair, with sitting time gradually increased to several hours a day. Depending on the size and weight of the patient and the kind of bed he is in, a bed-to-chair lift may be used to lift him mechanically from bed to chair. This may be scary for the patient, who needs to be reassured that the staff has been instructed in proper lifting techniques and that the procedure is safe. Once the patient becomes stronger, he will be taught simple, safe ways to get out of bed with little or no help. This technique is called a *transfer*.

Family and friends are encouraged to participate in increasing the patient's mobility. This is best accomplished by following the therapist's directions and encouraging the patient to move more independently every day.

Activities of daily living (ADL) are the things a person does throughout the day: homemaking, work-related tasks, recreation and play. The disruption of ADLs after a burn injury leads to a loss of independence. To help a patient regain function, the burn team will encourage the patient to do as much as possible on her own. Activities might include turning the television on and off, dressing, and assisting in simple wound cleansing and bandaging. Activities such as eating, brushing one's teeth and hair, or opening mail, which are simple under normal circumstances, are often strenuous for the burn patient and can be used as exercises. Activities can often be modified so the patient can do them more easily. For example, handles of eating utensils can be built up to compensate for a temporary decrease in hand motion (Figure 4.4).

A patient who is able to use his injured extremities to perform ADLs from the beginning of his burn unit stay will have a signifi-

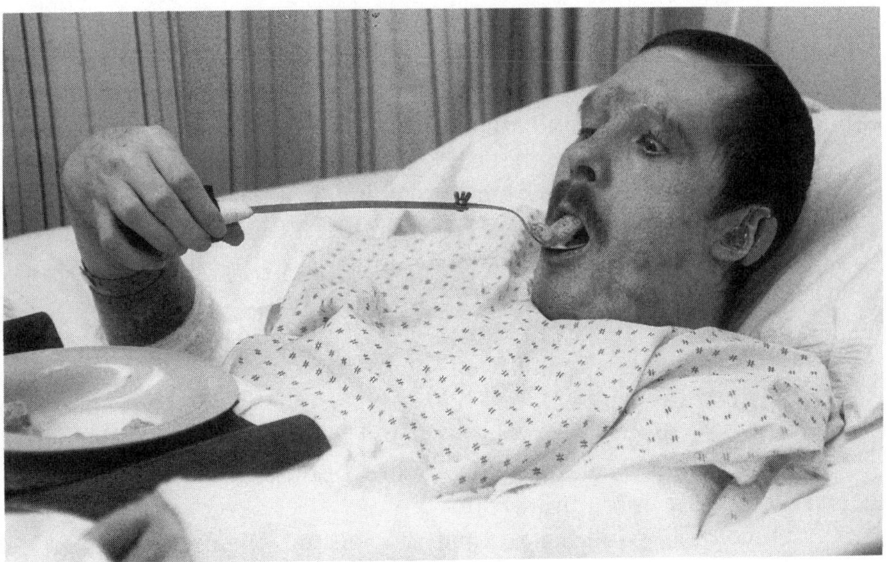

Figure 4.4. Adaptive devices are helpful for patients who are not quite ready to use everyday eating utensils.

cant increase in functional ability. As range of motion and strength increase, the need for adaptive equipment decreases. The more the burn survivor can do on his own, the better he will feel.

Walking

Most people take *ambulation*, or walking, for granted, but this essential skill can be lost after burn injury. Several factors must be taken into account when deciding whether an individual with a burn injury can or should walk. These include the ability to walk prior to the injury, the burn size, depth, and burn location, current burn-related medical problems, and current burn-related surgical procedures. The goal is for individuals to be able to walk as they did prior to the burn injury. The procedures outlined in this section apply generally to burn patients, although individuals who had problems walking before the burn injury are special cases and will require special attention.

At home

For individuals whose burn injury does not require admission to a hospital, the location and depth of the burn are the only factors that might limit ambulation. It is common practice to place patients with second-degree burns below the knee on bed rest, for example, to minimize additional tissue damage caused by the bursting of fragile capillaries in the wound. (The capillaries are tiny, thin-walled tubes that carry the blood between the smallest arteries and veins; they can be broken by the high blood pressures generated below the knee while standing.) Swelling induced by gravity can slow the healing of a wound, too, so the patient may be placed on bed rest to avoid this complication.

Being practical, we can see that even these individuals may need to walk at home—to and from the bathroom, to the kitchen for food, or to answer the door. This type of activity should be kept to an absolute minimum, however. Bed rest with the burned leg elevated on pillows, along with proper wound care, will help promote healing and minimize discomfort.

Once the wound has substantially healed, the individual can return to normal walking. Some individuals may begin walking without assistance, but others may require therapy for *gait training* (training to achieve a normal pattern of walking) and physical conditioning (see below). Individuals who do not have burns below the knee and are treated at home should be encouraged to be out of bed and walking. Maintaining as normal a daily routine as possible will improve the individual's overall recovery.

In the hospital

For the person admitted to the hospital with a burn injury, the factors mentioned at the beginning of this section can come into play. Regardless of the overall burn size, patients who have no burns below the knee and no other medical or surgical reason for bed rest should be out of bed and walking as much as they can tolerate. This helps maintain the patient's overall physical condition and promotes independence. Patients with second-degree burns below the knee are placed on bed rest and treated as described above. Patients with third-degree burns below the knee require skin grafting. No further damage can be done to the skin by walking prior to grafting, and since most patients are put on bed rest following the graft procedure, walking before the procedure is advised to retain physical conditioning up to the time of surgery.

The length of time bed rest is required following a below-the-

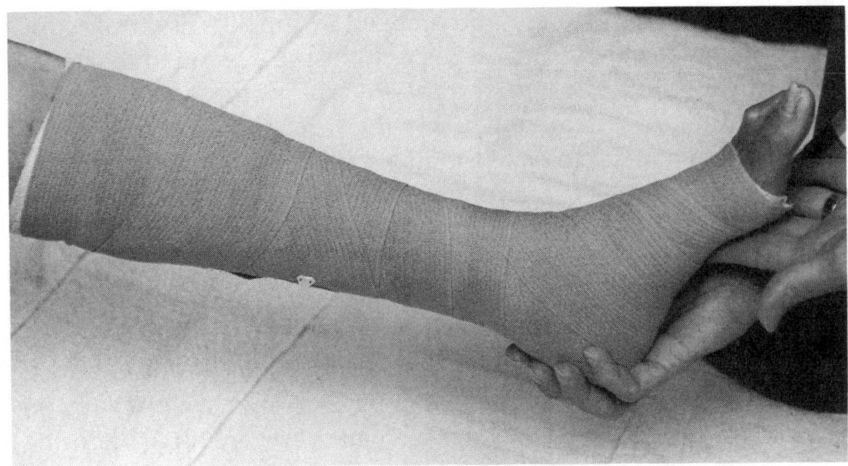

Figure 4.5. The Unna boot is designed to provide even compression and wound-healing medications when the patient begins to walk.

knee skin graft varies. Some physicians require their patients to remain immobile for up to 10 days following surgery, but the trend is to get the patient out of bed and walking as soon as it is medically possible. This rapid mobilization helps to decrease the incidence of certain complications and speeds the patient's return home.

For small, isolated burns below the knee that require grafting, some physicians apply a special supportive dressing in the operating room and allow the patient to walk the same day. Others wait from one to three days after surgery to apply these dressings and then initiate the walking. These supportive dressings consist of a layer of nonstick material placed directly over the fresh grafts, followed by the application of an Unna boot. The Unna boot is a roll of fine-mesh gauze that has been covered with a sticky paste of zinc oxide and calamine solution. This roll is applied to the leg, beginning at the toes and wrapping the leg up to the knee, to completely cover the grafts. A roll of dry gauze is applied over the Unna boot, and an elastic wrap is applied over the gauze. This dressing, which can be left on for several days, provides excellent support to the grafts and eliminates the need for daily dressing changes (Figure 4.5). Usually by six or seven days after surgery the Unna boot can be removed. Then only the elastic wrap need be worn by the patient while walking.

For patients who are not wrapped in supportive dressing for walking but who remain on bed rest, the progression to walking is a two-step process. First the patient will go through a *dangling* procedure to determine whether the regenerating circulation to the new graft can tolerate the added stress of ambulation. In this procedure the leg is carefully wrapped in an elastic bandage and then the patient is placed in a sitting position, with the leg hanging down, for slowly increasing time periods (usually one, two, and three minutes). Following each trial the leg is elevated, the elastic bandage is removed, and the graft is inspected for bleeding, breakdown, swelling, or color change (it should continue to look pink and should not be dark red or purple). The therapist will also ask the patient if she experienced pain or severe tingling during dangling (mild tingling that disappears quickly after the leg is reelevated is acceptable). If the patient has no problem following dangling, she will begin walking with the supervision of a therapist.

For patients with inhalation injuries who remain on a ventilator for a long period, and for patients who have severe medical complications or who have undergone multiple grafting procedures, the return to walking may be more difficult. For these patients the therapist either may attempt to maintain the individual's walking skills between procedures or may wait until medical complications are overcome. In these cases, ambulation may begin at the bedside or from a chair, with the therapist working initially with the patient on standing up and progressing to walking.

Sometimes walking is initiated in the rehabilitation clinic, using the parallel bars for stability and safety. The use of assistive devices such as walkers, crutches, or canes may be necessary for the patient to walk safely outside the parallel bars. Eventually the patient progresses to independent walking. For patients with severe limitations in walking, a wheelchair may be appropriate at discharge but should be discarded as soon as the therapist determines that the individual has made sufficient progress.

In the rare case of amputation involving the foot or leg, every effort will be made to help the patient progress to walking with a walker or crutches. A speedy transition to fitting and training with an artificial limb will help the patient's overall rehabilitation.

Once the patient has begun to walk on his own, the therapist will begin to teach the proper gait pattern. This includes walking with the head and trunk erect (rather than in a more comfortable bent position), with proper trunk rotation, and with bilateral arm swing (one arm forward, one arm back). The therapist will also teach the patient to put equal weight on each leg, to use the heel-toe pattern of walking, and to bend and straighten the hips and knees properly. The patient will gradually increase the walking distance and speed. Patients are taught to go up and down stairs and to negotiate ramps and curbs. If necessary, the patient will also be retrained to run, hop, jump, and skip.

Controlling Hypertrophic Scarring

Patients who have deep second-degree burns that heal without grafting, and patients who have burns that require skin grafting, are at risk of developing *hypertrophic scar tissue*. This tissue, which is thick, raised, and hard, may cause both functional and cosmetic problems that can delay or limit the patient's physical rehabilitation. One of the roles of the burn therapist is to control hypertrophic scarring.

The most critical factor in controlling the scar is the early and continued use of pressure. To be effective, pressure must be applied consistently to all deep burn areas and must be equivalent to at least 25 millimeters of mercury per square inch. Pressure therapy should begin as soon as the skin is healed and begins to feel dry. It should continue until the scarring process stops (until the scars reach maturity) and no further raising occurs. This is at least one year for adults and sometimes even longer for children.

The most effective way to provide adequate pressure is to use specially made elastic garments such as gloves, knee-length stockings, full-length tights, long- and short-sleeve vests, and face masks (Figure 4.6). Jobstskin, Barton-Carey, and Bioconcepts are three brands of commercially manufactured elastic garments. Each garment is individually measured so that all burned areas receive consistent pressure. Measurements can be taken before the patient leaves the burn unit or during an early clinic visit; garments usually arrive about two weeks later.

The garments must be worn as often as possible to be effective. Most patients wear their garments 23 hours a day, with time out

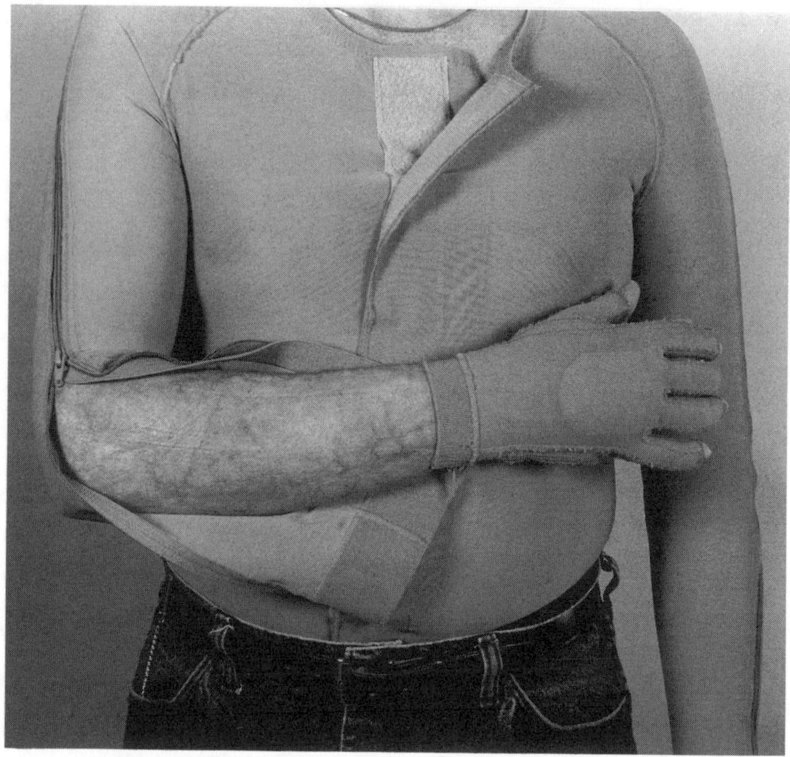

Figure 4.6. Garments designed to provide gentle compression of scar tissue are essential to control scarring. The more faithfully the garment is worn, the better the result.

only for bathing, and most patients have two sets of garments (one to wash and one to wear). With proper washing, drying, and care the garments usually last about 6 to 12 weeks, after which they must be replaced. The garments can be expensive, but their cost is generally covered by insurance and medical assistance programs.

Wearing pressure garments takes some getting used to. Even though the burns are healed, the skin is still tender and sensitive, and garments may be tight or may rub. If the garments cause skin breakdown, steps are taken to protect the areas where this occurs. After several washings the garments become softer and easier to wear. After the initial adjustment period many survivors report that they feel better when they are wearing the garments and describe them as a "second skin." The therapist can be helpful in answering questions and otherwise helping the patient during the adjustment phase.

Sometimes the patient is ready for pressure but the skin is too fragile to tolerate the elastic garments or the garment is not yet available. In these cases, other forms of pressure must be used. The simplest is an elastic bandage wrapped in a figure-eight pattern over the burn area. Depending on the body area, different sizes can be used, including 1-inch bandages for fingers. Tubular cotton elastic gauze (Tubigrip) is also used, because the cotton and rubber material is soft and more comfortable to wear. Because they can fit over a dressing, these bandages can often be used before the wound is completely healed. The tubular gauze is available as a prefit garment (including gloves) or on rolls. Its size varies to fit body parts from a small finger to a large trunk. The disadvantage of the tubular gauze is that it is not as durable as the custom-fit garments and easily stretches and frays.

For hands, Isotoner gloves may be used for early scar prevention. These gloves are like those that are available in stores, but they are not embellished by leather. They are turned inside out to prevent the seams from irritating tender skin. The fingertips of the glove are often removed to allow the person to feel things more easily and manipulate objects.

Web spacers may be worn between the fingers under the gloves for additional pressure to prevent scarring in this area, which may interfere with the person's ability to spread his fingers apart and move his thumb away from his hand. Web spaces are devices made of soft foam that fit into the web spaces between each finger and between the thumb and the index finger. Web spacers usually do not interfere with function.

There are times when additional pressure must be applied to specific areas. This may be accomplished by using Elastomer molds and Otoform and Silastic Gel Sheets. These molds and sheets conform to the scar tissue and are worn under the pressure garments. They must be removed periodically to check the skin and care for the skin. Some patients experience skin irritations or allergies, sometimes as a result of moisture accumulation. In most cases this irritation can be eliminated by removing the devices and washing and thoroughly drying the skin. Powder may also be applied to the skin to absorb excess moisture.

The complex contours of certain body areas present unique challenges in the application of pressure. For the face, custom-made elastic masks are available but often do not apply consistent pressure, particularly over the nose and around the mouth and eyes. The mask is difficult to put on and can frighten uninformed individuals who see the burn survivor wearing it. One solution is the custom-made transparent face mask and neck splint. These not only provide compression but also assist in preserving the natural contour of areas around the eyes, the mouth, and the Adam's apple.

The transparent splint is made in the following way. First, a negative impression of the face or neck is taken. (Ideally this is done when all swelling has subsided.) The impression is made by pouring GelTrate (a dental impression material) over the face or neck and then laying on plaster strips. When the material has hardened, it is removed and used to form a positive plaster cast. This is then sanded smooth, especially over areas with raised hypertrophic scar. The clear plastic material (W2) is heated in an oven and stretched over the finished plaster cast. Final adjustments are made to ensure that appropriate pressure is applied to scarred areas. Making the masks is the responsibility of the occupational therapy team.

Adequate pressure will cause the scar tissue to blanch, or turn white, and this can be observed through the plastic. The mask is held in place with soft strapping. Like all pressure garments, the mask must be worn as much as possible but can easily be removed for cleaning and skin care. The transparent masks may require frequent adjustments to improve compression as scar tissue changes. Adjustments can easily be made by filing and sanding the plaster mold and spot-heating the plastic mask.

Tightness of the mouth frequently occurs with facial burns when scar tissue forms around the corners of the mouth (called the *oral commissures*). This can interfere with the burn survivor's speech and ability to eat. A *mouth retractor* can be used to stretch the scar. A mouth retractor can be custom-made from splinting material. Or a prefabricated spring-loaded device can be purchased.

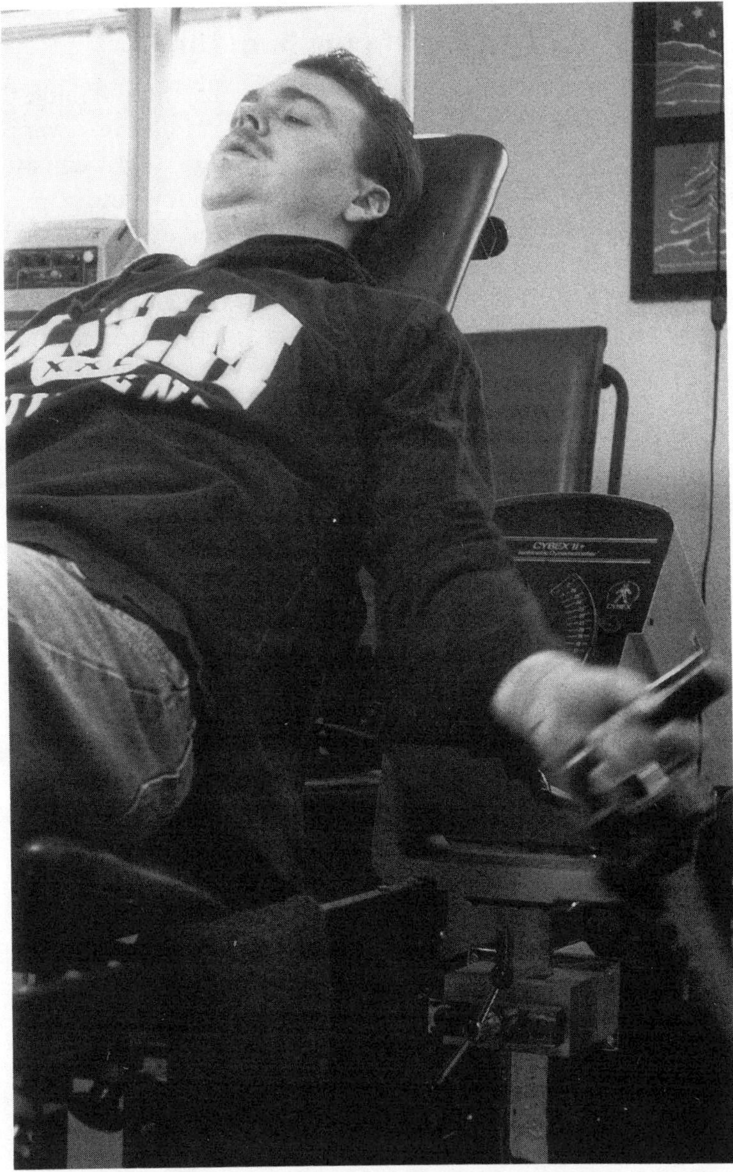

Figure 4.7. Exercise does not stop when the patient leaves the hospital. In fact, this is just a beginning. Continuing a regular program of exercise after discharge is essential for healing, recovery, and well-being.

After Leaving the Burn Unit

Before the patient is discharged to go home, the rehabilitation team will instruct the burn survivor and his family in a comprehensive home program. A daily home routine might consist of activities involving wound care, exercise, walking, and scar control. The therapists back up their verbal instructions by watching the patient and her family perform the activities by themselves before they leave the unit. The therapist also gives the patient individualized written and illustrated instructions to take home.

After the patient leaves the hospital, arrangements must be made for follow-up physical and occupational therapy. Patients who require more intensive therapy may need to go to an inpatient rehabilitation facility, and some patients may need nursing home care. If the patient is not able to leave his home frequently, a visiting therapist may be able to provide treatment in the home.

Most patients will receive follow-up therapy as an outpatient at the rehabilitation department of the burn center hospital or at a facility closer to the patient's home (Figure 4.7). Initially the patient may need to attend therapy on a daily basis, but treatment frequency can be reduced as the patient regains function. The burn center therapist will assist the patient and family in making the best rehabilitation choice and in arranging for the treatment.

Chapter 5

Psychosocial Rehabilitation

The personal experiences recounted in this book provide all the information that is needed to understand what a burn survivor has endured. Through these stories we learn about the trauma of the burn injury and the often difficult decisions made to survive, as well as the excruciating pain of the burn and the torture of dressing changes and physical and occupational therapy. The survivors describe their love-hate relationships with nurses and therapists; the long and often frustrating recovery and rehabilitation periods; the depths of loss, depression, and emotional upheaval; the immense changes in life roles and expectations; and the effect of the trauma on the family. These stories vividly illustrate how trauma indelibly alters the lives of the survivor and his or her close associates.

Each survivor is unique, and the journey through the burn unit and back into life has a richness that deserves individual attention and understanding. The following material is offered to help patients and family members better understand some of the complexities of that journey. (Psychosocial issues that are especially relevant to the recovery of the child burn survivor are taken up at the end of the chapter.)

The Experience of Trauma

We all would prefer that life events be predictable and, as much as possible, within our control. Gaining control of life events so that we can reliably meet our basic needs and avoid danger gives us a sense of personal safety and power. As our search for predictability and control progresses, some of us become stoic, unflappable individuals, and others become excitable, sensitive, and reactive beings. Likewise, some become extroverted, active, and high-spirited, while others are more introverted, reserved, and somber. Depending upon individual style and personality, each of us develops a certain degree of tolerance for ambiguity, stress, and change in our daily life as well as for the loss of predictability and control that results.

Initiating and maintaining satisfying relationships contributes to our view of the world as a safe and predictable place. The level of intimacy in our relationships with family and friends influences how much stress or change we can tolerate and is dependent to a great degree on our personal style. But everyone to some degree defines who he is by the amount and type of contacts he has with family and friends. Previous and current stressful experiences (for example, those relating to interpersonal relationships and to work) are also influential in the development of personality and coping skills.

Before a traumatic event, then, the individual has both a distinctive personality style and coping skills that work well for her. Based on her values, interests, goals, and motives, the individual makes certain assumptions about how and why the world works the way it does (this is her world-view). She uses her coping skills and contacts with friends to help her survive the difficulties she encounters and to make sense of and maintain adequate control of her environment.

The survivor

The traumatic event, by definition, stresses the individual on one or more levels. Physical tolerances may be breached, and emotional and cognitive coping skills may be overwhelmed by the intensity, severity, and duration of the stress. Furthermore, social networks may be damaged or broken through loss or estrangement. The sum of all these processes may threaten the person's world-view so that the person feels that the world is no longer safe or predictable.

The objective characteristics of the trauma—its severity, intensity, and duration—as well as the degree of damage and suffering it causes set the stage for the dynamic adjustment process that follows. The more intense the stress and the longer the stress exists, the more difficult adjustment is likely to be. Likewise, the greater the loss, the more difficult psychosocial recovery will be.

The better adjusted the individual is physically, emotionally, socially, and in the occupational and recreational arenas before the injury, the more likely he is to adapt adequately after the traumatic incident. Survivors who have a relatively high tolerance for ambiguity, change, and stress will be better able to manage the trauma and the treatment and rehabilitation that follow. A stable and supportive circle of family and friends also increases the likelihood that the individual can cope with the trauma. Finally, if the survivor believes that acceptable levels of control, judgment, and responsibility were exercised by himself and others during the trauma, he will be able to avoid strong feelings of shame or rage which can complicate adjustment.

Trauma and stress also often erode or destroy the very foundation of our lives in ways that may or may not be perceived as a loss by those who observe us. When we think of loss, loss of property and loss of life probably come to mind first. People may say to a burn survivor, "Well, at least you're still alive. Why should it bother you so much?" In fact, our appearance and our ability to perform tasks profoundly affect the core of our being. An interruption or loss of our ability to work, to socialize, or to have fun can also be devastating.

Severe trauma may challenge our belief that the world is safe and predictable, or that we can reliably obtain and keep what we value and need most. Injury can lead to a sense of vulnerability which makes a return to "normal" functioning very difficult to achieve.

Those close to the survivor

There is a growing recognition that trauma impacts those closest to the individual (family and friends) as well as the survivor. The survivor functioned within a circle of family, friends, neighbors, and co-workers prior to the trauma. Disruption of these relationships, whether temporary or permanent, affects all these people. And witnessing the traumatization of a person we care about often seriously affects us and can even produce secondary traumatization.

The traumatic event may challenge the family's basic need for predictability and control and contribute to a sense of vulnerability, even for those who were not directly involved in the incident.

The survivor and close associates alike may experience depletion of physical reserves. Uncertainty, worry, and disruption of routines change the rhythm of daily existence and may interfere with the relationships and roles of everyone involved. Added to the family's concern over the physical survival of the patient are financial, work, home, and child care concerns, all of which may be directly affected by the survivor's at least temporary inability to participate.

In the long run, the patients and families who do best seem to achieve a good balance between a strong sense of togetherness (cohesiveness) and a healthy respect for the need for the patient to share responsibility (autonomy). As one survivor said, "I knew I was pretty much back to normal when my wife began treating me like she always used to and no longer like a 'sick' person." The wife once again expected the patient to do the things around the house that he was responsible for. This couple had a strong feeling of togetherness through the trauma and the ordeal of recovery. This feeling is crucial early in the recovery phase; later on, the survivor's gradual resumption of normal activities and responsibilities becomes more helpful.

Understanding the likely course of recovery—both psychological recovery and physical recovery—benefits patients and families alike. Discussing psychological recovery in terms of stages (see below) can be helpful in the recovery process. Survivors and others who are familiar with these stages know what they can expect. It helps them to know what the different stages are, what the purpose of each stage is, and what can be done to address the needs of a person who is involved in any one of these stages of recovery.

The Stages of Recovery[1]

Both survivors and those close to them go through certain fairly predictable stages in postburn recovery and rehabilitation. During the hospitalization and immediate rehabilitation phases, the first five aspects of recovery tend to dominate. The last two take on greater significance as time goes on. Most people experience these phases to one degree or another, but some people experience one

[1] This section is adapted with permission from Watkins, Cook, May, and Ehleben, 1989.

or more stages and nothing at all of the others. Many survivors describe cycling through some stages on a regular basis for several years after the burn injury, while other people seem to progress smoothly through each stage.

Trauma brings about certain physiological changes known as the "fight or flight" response. This response lasts as long as the situation is perceived to be an emergency. The heart beats faster, breathing is faster and more shallow, blood flow to the muscles increases, and both excretion and digestion slow down. In the short run this response prepares the body to assess danger more accurately and to respond to it more quickly by running (flight) or combating it (fight). This response is very useful in responding to the burn incident.

The perception of danger and the physiological arousal just described can often continue in burn patients after the emergency is over, however. This leads to depletion of physical and emotional reserves, robbing the survivor of energy needed for the healing process. Part of the reason for this is psychological. The mind responds to trauma and painful stimuli as a narcissistic injury. This means that our basic sense of the invulnerability and integrity of our body and our personality is damaged. Some people respond to this damage in a fearful way; they become hypervigilant and apprehensive, and they avoid reminders of the burn incident. Other people become enraged; they are irritable and argumentative.

Fear and rage are adaptive reactions to trauma and often prevent further damage. When the source of discomfort is therapeutic, however, such as dressing changes or physical or occupational therapy, these emotional reactions usually prevent progress and may lead to further problems. Even further down the road, when distress is created by the emotional challenge of reentering society with a changed appearance and set of abilities, a different set of coping skills is required. These ideas are addressed in more detail below.

Survival anxiety

In this stage, the focus of concern is whether physical survival is possible. Symptoms of anxiety are common: hypervigilance and hyperventilation, sleep disturbances, an easy startle response, difficulty concentrating or remembering, disturbing dreams and memories of the injury, and depression. During this period, the patient and family should leave the day-to-day wound care to the burn team. For the patient and family to manage their anxiety, rage, and despair while remaining available to one another is paramount.

Survival is a realistic fear in the case of severe burn injury. Emotional and physical contact with loved ones plays a crucial role in the patient's physical recovery, but sometimes death is unavoidable. When the prognosis is grim, family, friends, and medical team need to respect the wishes of the mortally wounded and do everything possible to preserve that person's dignity. Some people in this condition request that only "comfort care" be given. Recognizing the likelihood of death, they choose to be allowed to die and only want treatment that is designed to manage the pain. Other patients request that all possible treatment be given, as they have decided to fight for survival, against the odds. If the person understands his medical situation and the various therapies available to him, and if his decision is his own, then either of these approaches is responsible, within our understanding of informed consent. Talking the situation over with medical, surgical, mental health, and pastoral counseling staff members can help the patient and the family make the best decision for them and accept the decision they make.

Following the death of a loved one, it will take time for the wounds of loss and grief to heal. Mood swings, lack of energy and appetite, and sleep disturbances are to be expected, at least temporarily, following the loss of someone close. The bereaved should try to be with other people, to share at least in this way the intensity of what they are experiencing. Over time they'll need to try to find words to talk about their emptiness and their search for the healing that will begin.

Even when the patient's chances for survival are good, worry about death will occur. This is a natural consequence of coming into contact with a life-threatening event. People who allow themselves to feel this anxiety, to talk about it and ask for appropriate clarification, will find their distress gradually relieved. Appointing one person in the family as the person responsible for obtaining information from the staff will reduce communication problems and help everyone receive information more quickly.

At this point the patient may be confused, groggy, anxious, or depressed. These are most likely temporary changes due to fever, pain medication, or traumatization, and they will lessen gradually over time. Calm, reassuring interactions in which the state of injury and treatment are realistically portrayed are much appreciated by the patient, who should be as involved as possible, even at this early stage, in making decisions regarding care, surgery, and so on. This involvement will help to restore a sense of control to the patient.

People who are extremely agitated after burn injury may also be given medication that has a calming effect. Systemic infections are often accompanied by high fever and delirium, causing the person to hallucinate—to see or hear things that are not really there—or to have thought disorders, imagining, for example, that people are relating to him in a strange way. Physical agitation may accompany these distressing mental activities. Antipsychotic medications provide relief from visual and auditory hallucinations and other thought disorders, and physical agitation may be treated with antianxiety medication. Physical restraints may be used if necessary to keep the patient from accidentally hurting himself or someone else. Sometimes it is necessary to use a paralyzing agent such as Pavulon to immobilize someone whose confusion and agitation are causing him to interfere with his own care. Unless the person had a psychological problem before the accident (which is likely to worsen under the stress of injury), however, the distressing symptoms of agitation will resolve when the cause of the delirium is addressed.

During the survival stage, family and friends often establish a vigil with rotating "shifts" in order always to have someone close to the patient. This is a good way to meet the needs of both patient and family. The shifts should be short in order to avoid wearing down the support group members. If they get sick and cannot function adequately themselves, they will not be able to help the patient at all. Family members especially need to allow others to share the burden and take time out for themselves periodically to restore energy and to remain engaged in their own support system.

Pain

The perception and experience of pain dominate our awareness until the pain is alleviated. As a species we could not have evolved if we did not escape pain and seek pleasure. Likewise as individuals, our training teaches us to limit painful experiences and to increase pleasurable ones. Patients in pain will grimace, brace themselves, be irritable and complain; they will request medication and apprehensively avoid activities that may increase the discomfort. Anxious vigilance for further signs of pain and depressive reactions to suffering dominate the mood. These emotional and behavioral reactions to the pain may actually increase the level of pain experienced.

The gate control model of pain seems to illustrate fairly well the factors that increase our perception of pain as well as how pain can be managed (Table 5.1). In this model we can see why both drug and psychological interventions are of value. The "gate" is the part of our physiology which determines whether the painful stimulation will reach our conscious awareness. It can be closed by several means. Medications are of greatest value in closing the gate at the physical sensation points by numbing pain sites, blocking pain signals to the brain, or helping us forget the past pain we have experienced. Cognitive and emotional factors work in a different fashion to close the pain gate. Because the human mind has the capacity to focus on only a limited number of things at any one time, we can use our emotions and our mind to focus our awareness on something pleasant, or to distract our attention from the pain, and thereby shut the gate.

Early on, when tissue damage is greatest and active healing continues, medication is the most important tool in managing pain. Cognitive and emotional factors are useful as adjuncts in enhancing the effect of the medication. In the first stages of recovery, pain medication must be adequate. There is no danger of addiction if medication is used for pain relief. Pain medication is *not* helpful and addiction *is* possible if pain medication is used to relieve anxiety or depression, however. Patients and those close to them need to recognize the differences between pain and other symptoms. While anxiety and depression can increase the percep-

Table 5.1. Managing Pain

	Factors That Open the Gate	Factors That Close the Gate
Cognitive/Evaluative	Worries Hypervigilance	Distraction Focusing
Emotional/Motivational	Fear Anxiety Depression	Calm Relaxation Involvement
Stimulation/Sensation	Tissue damage Scar Tissue	Massage Medication Warmth Coolness Movement (Differs by patient, type of injury, and stage of recovery)

tion of pain, they do not cause pain—nor are they relieved by pain medications.

Later, the emotional and cognitive skills of focusing and distracting attention and emotionally connecting with events outside the pain experience become more important, and pain medication is tapered off. Riveting attention on pleasurable and interesting activities or other aspects of the environment which can shut out awareness of discomfort is very beneficial. The survivor needs to take pain control as a serious personal challenge, because wound care and rehabilitation are uncomfortable, and progress can be impeded if adequate coping skills are not developed. Some patients focus on talking about things at home. Others focus on television shows or movies. Some become involved in games like checkers. Focusing mental powers on problems such as arithmetic or word games can also help. Distraction can also be provided by listening to music (Walkman radios may be especially soothing), reading, and talking with visitors. Progressive muscle relaxation and diaphragmatic breathing exercises decrease physiological arousal and increase the person's ability to focus on pleasurable distractions.

Pain often intensifies during such procedures as debridement, dressing changes, and physical therapy. Patients who manage pain effectively at these times generally use two strategies. The first is to distract their attention by focusing on another stimulus such as internal imagery or conversation or music from the environment. This seems most useful in closing the "gate" so that less pain is consciously perceived. The second strategy is to take on as much control of the painful stimulation as permissible (for example, by washing oneself or by doing range-of-motion activities on one's own). This seems to provide benefit by giving the individual a sense of predictability and control over when the discomfort takes place, how much discomfort there is, and how long the discomfort lasts.

Those close to the survivor can contribute by providing distraction and soothing interactions, by listening with concern to repetitive complaints, and by recognizing and encouraging all signs of self-management of pain.

Searching for meaning

The patient has a need to make sense of the injury and the circumstances surrounding the injury. This becomes the focus after survival is more secure and pain is adequately controlled. During this time patients often have nightmares, experience sleep problems, and relive disturbing memories of the accident. The desire to live in a safe and predictable world in which we can get what we need is basic to us all. As noted earlier, trauma can affect our sense of security and control. To reestablish this, we must determine and acknowledge the cause of the injury, our role in it, and its implications for the rest of our life. Searching for a logical explanation of the event allows us to make life seem predictable and controllable again.

The patient might have many seemingly irrational thoughts and explanations at this point, as various ways of thinking about the event are tried on for size. Patients may express disbelief or seem to deny that the event occurred. They may deny having any personal responsibility when some actually exists, or they may take on too much responsibility when no personal liability exists (guilt or shame). The patient may have dozens of questions about why the event occurred at all, and particularly "why to me?"

Denial or projection of blame as well as shame, guilt, or rage may dominate the patient's emotional life.

The search for meaning is a crucial stage of psychosocial recovery. The patients who do best develop a realistic assessment of the degree of personal responsibility and control involved as well as the adequacy of their behavior in response to the trauma. The important element seems to be the match between an objective view of our control, responsibility, and behavioral adequacy on the one hand and our own subjective view on the other. People who feel good about these things have an easier time making sense of the incident and putting it in its place.

For example, one father was injured when he returned to the burning house to rescue his son who was trapped. He knew that he was responsible for his injuries, but they made sense to him because he was injured doing what he *wanted* to do. He was in control. People who believe that they did not perform as expected, and who actually did not, stand to learn a greater degree of self-responsibility from the consequences of their actions. For example, one teenager realized that he was burned because he had been drinking too much and had passed out. Over time, he was able to recognize, struggle with, and eventually control his alcoholism.

Problems arise when there is a mismatch between how we believe we perform and how we actually did perform. In this circumstance, shame, guilt, or rage emerge and develop into self-defeating emotional states that interfere with the process of making a reasonable assessment of the trauma, its meaning in our life, and the effect on our life of any loss or disfigurement. For example, one worker blamed himself for his injury when there was nothing he could have done to prevent it. Another example is the mother who was injured getting her son out of the burning house. When the son later died from his smoke inhalation injury, the mother had a very hard time accepting that she had done the best she could do to save her child. Discussing the event with family, friends, and possibly a psychiatrist or a psychologist can help people such as these develop a realistic view of the event. Then they will be better able to make an adequate adjustment.

Investment in recuperation

The patient can focus on treatment and rehabilitation more fully once survival is ensured, pain is controlled, and life again seems somewhat predictable and controllable. Personal responsibility for maximizing recovery of function and appearance is resumed. Upswings in mood and physical activity often occur at this point, and the patient begins to make plans for resuming as much of the old lifestyle as possible. The patient may begin to request feedback about her progress and may begin to compare herself with other patients at this time.

It is usually not advisable to force the burn survivor to acknowledge prematurely the degree or the finality of losses in his function or appearance out of a misguided desire to have the survivor "face the facts." As one patient pointed out, the hope for further improvement or even a complete return to preburn appearance and function "can be very useful in keeping you motivated to pursue reconstructive work and to endure the long hours, weeks and months of therapy." The somewhat unpredictable course of scarring and the role of motivation and effort in regaining functions make hope an important emotion.

A good rule is to let the survivor set the pace in accepting the degree of loss of appearance and function. An incomplete acknowledgment of the severity of the injury is functional in two ways. First, as noted above, it may help the person stay motivated and work harder in rehabilitation and follow medical regimens more accurately. Second, the emotional adjustment to impaired function or disfigurement can be made over time and thereby be made easier. Some severely injured patients have related that it took years after the injury before they could acknowledge that they had been permanently changed.

Acceptance of losses

The frustration of rehabilitation and the amount of effort and time it requires eventually help the survivor recognize how likely it is that he will have a loss of function and appearance. Frustration increases as the point of diminishing returns is approached. That is, there is a point at which further effort will have very little effect. From an objective view, there is a full range of loss—from minimal to almost total loss of function and appearance—but in fact, loss is subjectively experienced. What is minimal to one person may be perceived as a major loss to another, and what is major to one may seem minor to another.

During this stage, family and friends may notice depressed mood, self-absorption, sleep and appetite disturbance, and less activity by the patient. The patient may report loss of hope and may even question the value of life at this point. The greater the perceived disruption of preburn lifestyle, and the less likely the full return to that life, the more acutely the threat to self is experienced. Most burn survivors have these feelings to some degree. If the feelings interfere with the person's ability to function in certain roles or to enjoy life, however, or if they lead to thoughts of death or suicide, it is time to seek professional help.

It is helpful at this point for survivors and those close to them to recognize that the feelings of grief are legitimate; these feelings need to be experienced by the survivor, who also needs to express them to someone who truly cares and understands on an emotional level. Over and over patients emphasize the importance of emotional understanding and true caring about the depth of their pain. Realistic feedback about progress when requested by the patient is crucial, as are descriptions of realistic expectations for the recovery of function and appearance. Burn team members can help provide this information. The feedback must be appropriately timed, based on the survivor's readiness to hear it. Sincerity, honesty, concern, and consistency are needed from members of the social support system at this time.

This support is often most vital when the patient begins to look at and come to terms with the appearance of the wounds. In the early stages patients may ask for information about their appearance, but what they are really requesting is feedback that will allow them to judge the emotional impact of the wounds and scars *on the observer*. The best indication of a patient's readiness to begin to regain a sense of positive self-image occurs when the patient requests a mirror. Hopeful but realistic feedback about appearance and its impact on the viewer must be given before the patient looks in the mirror. This feedback must be given gradually, so the individual can build up to being able to tolerate the feelings that the sight of the wounds or scars will arouse in himself and the viewer. Members of the burn care team are often the best source of realistic expectations regarding appearance. They have a wealth of experience with wounds of various sizes, severity, and locations and can give good estimates of the eventual appearance once wounds have healed and scars have matured. The need to tailor the pace of this feedback to the patient's readiness was expressed by one survivor, who said, "Changes in appearance can be extensive, and we all have our own ways of getting ready for becoming aware of this—and that needs to be respected."

Some burn survivors report having a much more intense experience when they view themselves in mirrors they are familiar with. The small mirrors and unfamiliar lighting in the hospital may cause the patient to minimize the changes in that setting; changes observed at home or work, however, where the patient has observed his reflection for years, may be more apparent and more difficult to deny. Family and friends need to be aware of this possibility and provide support to the survivor who is viewing himself in a familiar mirror and setting for the first time.

Investment in rehabilitation

The difficult challenge of recognizing and accepting our losses may be met gradually as we begin to define a new lifestyle and to recognize that this new lifestyle, though different, may be satisfying nonetheless. One patient who was facing for the first time the possibility of being wheelchair bound said he wouldn't want to live like that. Six months later, still uncertain about the outcome of surgeries and rehabilitation, his view had changed: "I guess you can get used to anything if you have enough time," he said. The passing of time helps, as does friendly support and the development of an interest in activities that are possible within the limits set by changed capabilities.

The patient's investment of time and effort in rehabilitation at this stage involves not only optimal recovery of appearance and function but also the pursuit of a full and satisfying lifestyle. This is when the survivor begins exploring to find out which aspects of pre-injury roles and functions can be resumed. For some people, this may be as easy as "getting back into the swing of things." The challenge may be greater for others and may actually involve developing an entirely new set of work, play, and familial and social roles and functions.

Most survivors seem to make progress first in the life areas that are most important to them and then turn to achieving gains in roles and functions that have secondary importance. For example, a survivor who derived great pride and pleasure in her work quickly progressed through physical rehabilitation early on and returned to the job. Only later did she work at becoming more comfortable in social situations where others might see her scars.

Reintegration of identity

Many survivors describe themselves as having begun a new life at the time of their injury. This is only partly because of changes in goals and activities. There is also a recognition that experiencing so much random destructive power and suffering through acute pain and enduring rehabilitation alters the way we approach, prepare for, and experience life.

The exploration by the survivor into roles and functions eventually affects his internal sense of self, sometimes resulting in a redefinition of gender identity, partnership, or parenthood. The final implications of traumatization and losses in function, appearance, or roles are also recognized. The needs, desires, goals, and values that were in place prior to the injury may need to be reexamined in light of the long-term and permanent losses sustained.

Survivors need to restore their sense of safety and order in the world and their sense of power and control. Family and friends can help this process by listening to the often repeated complaints of pain, fear, or rage and expressing concern over and understanding of what the survivor is experiencing. An important contribution of family and friends is recognizing and encouraging each step toward independence that the survivor is able to take. Eating on their own, calling the nurse, and sitting up are major accomplishments for many patients. No matter how small the step appears compared with what the person was able to do before the burn, each success must be applauded.

The challenge posed to one's identity after a major burn injury varies according to the nature of the injury and other factors. Some of these are discussed in the following section.

Life Areas Affected by Severe Burn Injury

Body function, appearance, and self-image

The physical functions most valued and most often used are those that have the greatest impact on self-image. This makes sense when we think about it: we use our eyes and our hands to interact with the world in one way or another almost every waking moment. Furthermore, in order to survive we must use our nose and mouth to breathe, drink, and eat. Likewise, we use our feet and legs to mobilize in the pursuit of our goals, we relate to others through what we hear, and we have an impact on others through our sexual arousal patterns, our external appearance, and what we say. One aspect of nearly every surface characteristic we have is directly related to such fundamental needs as obtaining and consuming food and water, establishing and maintaining social connections, and obtaining those pleasures that give life its variety and flavor.

The effect on the individual of functional loss and impairment has been discussed in earlier chapters. The point being made here is that surface characteristics form the foundation of many of the behaviors by which we define ourselves.

Gender is one of the qualities by which people identify themselves to themselves and to the world. Gender is declared through hair, makeup, and clothes and grooming as well as through a personal style of relating to persons of the same sex and persons of the opposite sex. Concerns about changes in appearance and changes in functional abilities can strike at the core of our sense of being attractive and lovable. Burn survivors are often called on to look deeper into themselves, and subsequently others, to ascertain the sense of beauty and worth that was formerly obtained by attention being paid to physical appearance. In the long run this can lead to a richer understanding of life and what it means to be a lovable and attractive human being. In the short run it can mean waves of grief, rage, anxiety, and depression as the realization of loss sinks in.

A patient's sense of herself as a sexual being may be impaired by a decrease in function or appearance. The skin is where intimate contact is made, and in order to fully experience physical and emotional pleasure we must be comfortable with both our own skin and appearance and that of our partner. For the burn survivor and her partner, many factors can interfere with this comfortable interaction. Some patients withdraw from physical contact for fear of being rejected by the other, and some patients only passively accept the advances of the other, refusing to "give" as well as "take." This may be the result of feeling less lovable and attractive as a result of a changed appearance.

Partners may have their own difficult emotional reactions to work through. Fear of damaging or hurting the survivor, fear of causing embarrassment, and fear of revealing one's own inhibitions about touching damaged skin all may come into play. The strong, mutual relationship the survivor and the partner used to share may be damaged as one or the other becomes less of a peer and more of a caretaker, afraid to express his or her own needs and desires for fear of burdening the other.

The burn trauma, dressing changes, and tubbings, as well as the stretching and straining of physical and occupational therapy, can also lead the patient to be awkward about, or even afraid of, skin exposure and contact. His changed appearance and changes in function and sensation may lead him to feel shame, fear, or other negative emotions that get in the way of intimacy. Furthermore, fear of infection is great in the burn unit, and many patients remain leery of infection even after wounds have closed. They may shy away from skin contact as a result.

One way many people recover from these conditions is to gradually increase contact with and exposure of the skin in an increasingly intimate manner. Early on in treatment, partners can learn how to cleanse and dress wounds. They may also massage the skin with soothing oils and creams. As rehabilitation progresses, massages become increasingly helpful as a way of loosening joints and returning sensitivity to the skin.

The nonverbal but nevertheless emotional communication of touch and massage can begin to heal internal wounds. Gradually finding the courage and the words to make requests and to express feelings will follow. Both survivor and patient will benefit if they focus on the pleasurable sensation of warmth and touch, allowing themselves to feel their passion. Looking into each other's eyes and whispering in each other's ears, partners usually find their hearts opening and mutual attraction growing as inhibitions and apprehensions diminish.

Relationships

Family, marital, sexual, and social relationships all play a major role in helping the survivor be comfortable with her appearance and gradually developing a deeper sense of worth. This is because people internalize what they experience externally. In other words, as we experience encouragement, understanding, challenge, and a return to normality in relating to others, we can begin to follow the same route for ourselves. The path can be a difficult one, however, and negotiating it requires consistency, communication, and honesty.

Friends and family can best relate to survivors by giving them emotionally honest feedback when they request it. It is important for the survivor to communicate directly and assertively as well. Both the survivor and those close to him need to be honest with themselves about the feelings brought on by the wound or scar. When the patient asks whether the sight and feel of the wound or scar are "okay," what the patient is asking is this: "Can you see that I am still here even though my appearance, and perhaps my abilities, have changed?" By talking about the appearance of the injury, by looking at the injury regularly for long periods of time, by letting the feelings of aversion come and go, both survivors and their loved ones can begin to see the internal beauty again.

A word about the aversion we sometimes feel when we look at wounds and scars and about our wish to stare at them or to look away. There is probably a primitive adaptive element in these behaviors. When we see something new in the environment, we look at it until we determine whether we are in danger from it or whether we will be comfortable having further contact with it. An unusual appearance in a person may be a sign of disease processes that endanger us, for example. People who have good social skills may be more adept at looking quickly and then looking quickly away, but they need to look nonetheless. Unfortunately, this need "to look" must be satisfied whether or not the survivor is comfortable with the changes in his appearance or having people see these changes. Because of this, the survivor should be the one setting the pace for gradual exposure to social situations where staring might occur.

As the survivor's tolerance for the changes in appearance develops along with that of his family and friends, so does the ability to tolerate the reactions of others. If the patient asks for an honest appraisal of the appearance of the wound, those close to him should make a direct and honest statement. On the other hand, anyone who feels a need to comment on the wound ought, really, to seek permission from the patient before doing so. Some people cope with stares from strangers by reminding themselves silently that "this person is being rude and I don't have to let him get to me." Others have found it useful to look away for a few moments when meeting new people. This allows the new people to stare, become comfortable with the scars, and regain their social amenities.

Work and leisure activities generally entail less intimacy than do family, marital, and sexual relationships, but they often help us define who we are. As discussed earlier, we are defined to some extent by the things we do most often and most consistently. For many of us, these are our habits of work and play.

The personality of the patient plays a major role in how the wound and scarring affect work and play. People who are sociable and place great emphasis on being with others and who are very sensitive to the emotions of others may be more greatly affected by the reactions of themselves and others to looking at and touching visible burn wounds and scars. People who experience their feelings more strongly and who derive great pleasure from being attuned to intellectual, emotional, and physical stimulation through cultural and aesthetic activities may also experience the impact of the injury to a greater degree. Those who are more individualistic, less involved with others, and less concerned with their own or others' reactions to the scarring may be affected less noticeably.

A good rule for the patient in terms of returning to school, work, and other regularly scheduled activity involving contact with others is to wait until she is able to tolerate her own reactions and the reactions of others. The "sink or swim," "let's do it all at once" schools of thought may work for some people but probably will not work for the majority of people. Goal setting (discussed below) may facilitate the return to work or school (see also Chapter 7).

Goal Setting

Sometimes it is useful to develop a systematic approach to reentering society, reestablishing intimacy, getting back to work, and broadening the pursuit of leisure activities. In general, the patient needs to set realistic goals that leave him with a sense of progress but which are neither too tough nor too easy. Setting sights too high or too low is to be avoided. Starting with relatively easy challenges and building up to more difficult ones is to be encouraged. Starting with those goals that involve less threat and more pleasure and working toward those perceived as more stressful or threatening is also to be encouraged, as is rewarding oneself after accomplishing each small step. Success breeds successes.

Some people like to group several challenges together in order to maximize the effect of their effort, just as other people prefer alternating periods of work with periods of rest so they can appreciate their progress and prepare for the next step. Some people may find it useful to anticipate setbacks and plan to attack a goal several times before succeeding. This may help keep setbacks from robbing them of the motivation to continue pursuing those goals that are most important. Requesting appropriate social support during each challenge and as a reward for effort may also prove beneficial for the survivor, family, and friends. Follow these guidelines when setting and working to achieve goals:

- Set goals that allow progress to be seen
- Share goals with people whose feedback you value
- Take active and manageable steps toward these goals
- Reward each accomplishment
- Assess progress made toward each goal while setting new goals or revamping original goals

Setting reasonable goals and acknowledging progress toward achieving them establishes a positive feedback loop. Each goal we meet should enhance our beliefs about personal power. This enhances self-esteem and, in combination with available skills, allows the person to actively pursue the things he values the most. This tests the concept many of us have that we lack the necessary power and control to achieve our goals. By taking a series of small steps we gain the feedback that shores up our sense of predictability and control, which is essential to our psychosocial recovery.

Getting Professional Help

A person who is having problems adjusting psychologically to the burn injury can benefit from structured short-term interventions, which are designed to teach the person about the healing process that takes place after traumatic loss and to provide training in methods of managing and alleviating symptoms. There are different kinds of interventions. You will need to decide what kind of professional to see, what modality of treatment to seek, and what strategy for recovery to follow.

Social workers, psychologists, and psychiatrists are all qualified to provide counseling, and so it is usually personal preference and need that determine which kind of professional a person sees. People who view their problems as being focused on areas of interpersonal relationships may prefer to go into counseling with someone who has expertise in group or family counseling. People who are anxious or depressed about trauma-related issues, on the other hand, might prefer to work with someone who is experienced in managing anxiety and depression and in helping the person recover a sense of control and self-esteem. The person whose self-image has been damaged by loss of function or changed appearance might do best seeking the help of a professional who is proficient in helping establish healthy attitudes toward changed abilities.

The *modality of treatment* refers to the setting of the counseling: individual, family, and group counseling are all options. A person generally chooses a modality of treatment based on personal comfort within a particular setting and the optimal *strategy* for recovery. People choosing to focus on disturbed family relationships through an interactive strategy might choose family counseling, while a person who chooses a medication strategy (treatment with antidepressant or antianxiety medications) usually meets with the counselor individually. People may choose to ease the torment of symptoms by learning new thought processes and behavioral responses though either group or individual modalities.

Psychological Rehabilitation for the Child

A stay in the hospital can be a tense experience for anyone. A child facing an unexpected hospitalization will encounter a variety of new experiences, including pain and separation from parents and family. The child's parents will face a multitude of questions: How will my child react to being in the hospital? What is the hospital staff going to do to my child? How can I help my child with the pain? Will I be able to help with my child's care? Can I be with my child all of the time? How am I going to keep my other children and family members together? What's going to happen when my child leaves the hospital? This section will address some of the issues, questions, and concerns that may arise during a child's hospitalization.

Frequently, when a child is burned, she is whisked away from her family and brought to the hospital by ambulance or helicopter. Usually parents cannot accompany the child, so the child begins the journey with an unfamiliar person. Even though this person will try to comfort and reassure the child, the first encounter after the burn injury is still with a stranger.

When the child arrives at the hospital, she will likely be taken immediately to the burn unit. Evaluation by the medical and nursing staff takes place, and then transportation to a regular or intensive care room, as the case demands. While in her room, the child will see many unfamiliar faces and may hear unfamiliar noises from machines in the rooms around her. The staff will reassure the child until the parent or caretaker can be reunited with her.

Parents may have many fears and feelings of anger, guilt, and anxiety during their child's hospitalization. The hospital staff remains available to work closely with the child and family members to provide education, to listen, and to lend support whenever needed.

Age-related problems from infancy to adolescence

Children's reactions to being in the hospital vary according to age. Infants (birth to six months of age) may appear unaffected psychologically by medical treatment as long as they are nurtured by a caring individual. If a child is separated from the parent at this time, the bonding and attachment process may be interrupted. This is usually much more difficult for the parent than for the baby, however.

As a child reaches the ages of 7 months to 18 months, she becomes aware of the permanence of objects and consequently fears separation. Any prolonged time away from family members at this period results in a feeling of abandonment. At this age it is important for family or caretakers to be as involved as possible in the child's care. If the child is in an intensive care setting, the parent may not be allowed to stay in the area all night, but when it is possible, parents should stay overnight. Children in this age group do not respond as well to health care workers as older children do and therefore will be more at ease with family members present.

Starting at about 18 months until 3½ years of age, a child does not see separation from parent and family as abandonment and does not become quite so anxious when his loved ones have to leave. Children in this age group may be more worried about no longer being lovable than they are that their parents have abandoned them. They may also view hospitalization as a punishment for misbehavior, or they may believe their illness was caused by something they did, like not eating or not listening. It is therefore crucial for the family and staff to continually reassure the child that they are not making the child stay in the hospital as a punishment but because the child is sick and being in the hospital will help her get better.

Children 3½ to 5 years become concerned with physical damage to their body. They fear any invasive procedure such as injections and dressing changes, and they need clear explanations of what is going to happen to them. Giving them an opportunity to work through their fears, using play, may help them overcome circumstances that frighten them in the hospital.

The school-aged child, 6 to 12 years, worries a great deal about missing school and the loss of socialization with peers. But his greatest fear is the loss of ability to make choices. It is important at this time to afford the child the opportunity to have some choices. This could consist of simple things like selecting meals, selecting activities, or choosing his own hospital attire, if possible. Allowing him to participate in his daily care (tubbing and dressing changes) can also provide the child with a sense of independence. For school-aged children as for other children, being honest and giving clear explanations of all procedures will lead to the development of positive, trusting relationships.

Adolescence is a particularly difficult psychological period.

Even more than most burn patients, adolescents need others to make every effort to meet their emotional and physical needs throughout their hospitalization. Some of the issues these young patients are concerned about are privacy (not necessarily a private room, but private space), having some control over their daily care, and peer socialization. Some of these needs can be met by allowing them to sleep late, to participate in or even do their dressing changes, to have their friends visit when possible, and to participate in fun activities. A great deal of patience is needed here, because a nurse can take a dressing off much faster than a child. But it's worth it. Giving adolescents some choices can lead to better cooperation.

Throughout the child's hospital stay, the parent may see behaviors or sense feelings that are new. The parents need to remember that the child may be scared, anxious, lonely, bored, and in a great deal of physical pain. These feelings can easily cause frustration and, sometimes, result in misbehavior (see Chapter 1, under "Pain").

Parental involvement in therapy

Hospitalization for a severe burn is a crisis for both the child and the family. Institutions try to ease the crisis in various ways. Although rules and regulations vary from hospital to hospital, many pediatric and other similar burn facilities offer options like parental rooming-in, pediatric meal choices, educational services, playroom and recreation area and staff, and sibling visitation. All these efforts to make the hospital environment pleasant and more "homelike" improve the child's chances for a quick, more positive, and less traumatic recovery.

Rooming-in may be available in general pediatric units but usually is not in intensive care settings. Some intensive care units provide a room or space where parents can spend the night, which is usually away from the child's room. But if the child is admitted to a unit that allows rooming-in, one parent may be able to stay and participate in the child's daily care and be there to reassure and support the child.

Parental involvement in feeding (providing encouragement and assistance) may be crucial, since nutrition is an important factor in the healing process of a burn. Offering foods from home or snacks the parent knows the child likes can aid in the healing process, physically and emotionally. (Parents need to check all foods in with the staff, in case the child's calories are being counted.)

Family involvement is encouraged. Sibling visitation, when permitted by the hospital, can improve the burn survivor's emotional well-being. Children who are hospitalized need to spend time with their brothers and sisters, and siblings of a child who has been burned may be worried about the child and may need first-hand reassurance that their brother or sister is getting better. Family support is terribly important, especially to a child who faces an extended hospitalization and multiple surgical operations.

Another way to create an atmosphere that is as "normal" as possible for the hospitalized child is to offer the child a chance for play and recreation, peer socialization, and relaxation. Children need to play and be as active as possible, and they need to move their burn-injured body part to reduce atrophy and contraction from disuse. If the child is able to get out of bed, either by walking or in a wheelchair, this should be encouraged. This will help the child feel more at home and enable him or her to be with other children who are sick and in need of companionship, reassurance, and attention. Peer socialization within the hospital setting can raise a child's spirits, increase motivation, and contribute to emotional and physical healing.

The use of medical play, with puppets or dolls, can help familiarize a child with hospital procedures and gives the child an opportunity to act out fears and anxieties about hospitalization in a play situation. If a child is not able to come to the playroom, activities may be provided in her room. The child life/play therapist is responsible for this activity.

Emotional support, school, and rehabilitation

A child who is going to be hospitalized for an extended period of time needs to do some schoolwork if possible, to maintain a sense of normalcy. Very often tutors are available within the hospital or will be sent from the school district. If a tutor is not available, having a classmate or teacher bring the work will help the child feel as if she is not falling behind and will give her a chance to keep in contact with her school friends. Schoolwork can increase the variety of activities the child engages in during the day, making the hospital experience more bearable.

There is no doubt that parents will see changes in a burned child's behavior during hospitalization and will need to be prepared to react with an appropriate emotional response. Children act, react, and interact differently when parents are present. They may be calmer and more relaxed, but quite often they are more demanding, even to extremes. It is very important for parents to listen to the child, give him reasonable choices, and support and nurture him—and also set limits when necessary. Even though the child is injured and in the hospital, limits need to be set, just like at home. Children have the ability to manipulate their parents and make them feel guilty while all along exhibiting inappropriate behavior. Parents who are firm but supportive and nurturing help both parents and staff to retain control when the child is acting out.

Throughout the child's hospitalization the staff will be available to support the parents, answer all questions, and help the parent better understand the child's hospital stay. When discharge is imminent, the staff will prepare the child and the family for the child's return to home and the community. If a child must go home with dressings, parents will be taught how to change and reapply the bandages, and a follow-up appointment will be made for the child and parents to return to see the burn team.

If the child goes to school, a school reentry program may be available (see Chapter 7). This program is set up and administered by hospital staff to educate the child's classmates and teachers about burns and burn treatment. It is designed to help the child feel more comfortable returning to school and community, and to help those in the school and community have a better understanding of burn injuries and prevention.

A children's support group can help meet social, recreational, and emotional needs. For burn patients who don't want to participate in groups, individual or family counseling can be arranged by hospital staff. Throughout the child's stay, and after her return home, the burn unit staff is available to answer questions and offer support to the child, the family, and the community. Many parents and patients have ongoing relationships with the hospital staff and other patients who help the child and the family continue on the road to recovery.

Summary

A person who is undergoing psychosocial rehabilitation after a burn injury will travel through a series of stages. The earliest involves physical survival, reduction of discomfort, and making certain that the trauma does not recur. Later the person addresses issues surrounding maximizing recovery of physical skills and functions or training in new ones. The progress he makes in these areas prepares him to begin to come to terms with the changes he has gone through and become whole again.

At this stage the person is prepared to accept herself with both her wholeness and her brokenness. When this is accomplished, she works at resuming social activities with family and friends and, eventually, resuming work and play activities. With this self-acceptance she can respond appropriately both to those who would shun her because of her injuries and to those who would treat her like an invalid because of her struggles.

The emotional journey to recovery is seldom a straight path. It is much more common to move in fits and starts, feeling great one day and hopeless the next. Taking one day at a time and having a clear plan as to what goals need to be achieved by what point in time is one way of staying on track. The person who remains aware of how far he has already come and who makes use of the people who can help him get where he wants to go is working in the right direction.

Chapter 6

Reconstructive Surgery

Burn injury disrupts the functions of the skin, the body's largest organ. These functions are crucial to the health of the body as a whole, and therefore early burn treatment is directed primarily toward replacing the body coverage that had formerly been provided by the skin. Reconstructive burn surgery, the subject of this chapter, takes place later and is largely dedicated to addressing and treating the problems that remain after the acute burn wound has healed. In this chapter we describe how reconstructive surgery and other treatments improve or correct the physical problems caused by burn injury.

The Healing Process

If left to heal spontaneously, the body will replace its skin cover through two primary healing processes: *epithelialization* and *contraction*. When epidermal skin cells (also called epithelial cells) lose contact with the cells that have been destroyed, the healthy cells divide, multiply, and move across the open wound to cover it. When the wound is superficial, this process—epithelialization—is the primary mode of healing, and the resulting scar is relatively minimal (Figure 6.1).

When the wound is deeper, healing elements of the epidermis may have been destroyed and therefore are not available for epithelialization. In this case the body closes the skin defect by drawing on the surrounding skin. This process of pulling the wound margins in toward the center of the wound is called contraction. Indeed, as the wound heals, it actually shrinks, or becomes smaller. Contraction is a natural process, the body's attempt to close the wound. But contraction can also cause deformities in

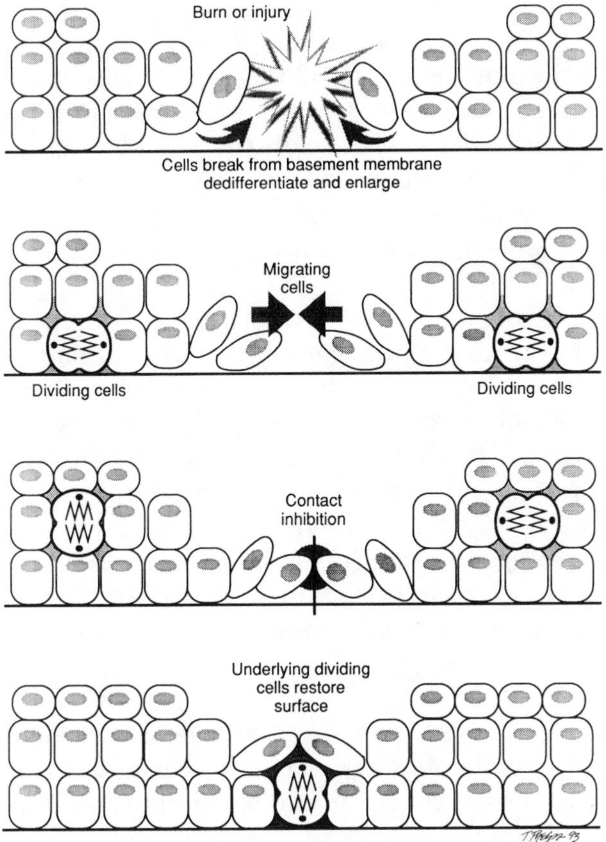

Figure 6.1. Epithelialization is the primary mode of wound healing for superficial wounds.

deep burn injuries, as the same process that leads to contraction of the wound can result in "heaping up" of the burn scar or in the formation of tight scar bands across joints which limit their function. When excess scar tissue accumulates, *hypertrophic scars* or *keloids* are formed. Scar bands that limit joint mobility are called *contractures*. Because they cause dysfunction or deformity, all of these scars are considered *pathological scars*.

In designing a treatment plan for a patient with a burn injury, physicians must use their best judgment to determine which wounds will heal spontaneously by epithelialization and which ones will heal not by epithelialization but by contraction. In wounds that heal by epithelialization, relatively acceptable scarring and healing result. In most partial-thickness and full-thickness wounds that are expected to heal by contraction, however, skin grafts will be used to close the wounds. As noted earlier in this book, it is difficult to assess the severity of the burn injury for several days after the injury occurs, and even the most experienced burn surgeons are unable to determine the depth of burn in every case.

Although skin grafts close the wound and save the life of the patient, they tend to continue to contract after healing, and they do not replace all of the functions of normal skin. Furthermore, because the split thickness of the skin grafts (only a portion of the dermis is removed with the epidermis) cuts across the sweat glands and hair follicles, these structures are not transferred with split-thickness skin. For these reasons, the split-thickness skin graft used in treating acute burns is frequently less than completely satisfactory as the final coverage in terms of the person's ability to move and the person's appearance.

Normal scar tissue

The body repairs itself by forming scar tissue. We can see scar tissue on the surface of the body, but scars also form under the surface of the body wherever destruction and repair of tissue has occurred.

When an injury first occurs, certain of the body's blood cells are attracted to the wound to help rid it of dead and damaged tissue, foreign substances (such as dirt), and any bacteria that may have entered the wound. This initial phase of healing lasts for five to seven days and is called the *inflammatory phase.*

Scar tissue is made up of collagen, a protein that is manufactured and deposited in the healing wound by a cell called a fibroblast. As the first phase of healing ends, fibroblasts migrate into the wound and start laying down collagen to form scar tissue. The scar that initially forms is often red, raised, and very thick. This second phase is called the *proliferative phase,* referring to the proliferation of collagen or scar tissue. Particularly during the first six to eight weeks after injury, a large amount of collagen is formed, resulting in thick scars.

Even as the collagen is being laid down, an enzyme called *col-*

lagenase begins breaking down the collagen. Although this process starts soon after injury occurs, only after two or three months does a balanced state develop, in which the amount of collagen being removed is equal to the amount of collagen being formed. We have all experienced the maturation of scar tissue, the phenomenon referred to as "fading." The stage in which the scar fades is known as the *maturation phase*; it can last up to two years following the injury. Physical and occupational therapies can effectively modify scars during this phase by applying external forces to the collagen as it is being built up and broken down, to make the new collagen more like the normal structure of the skin.

Although most scar tissue matures and becomes more like normal skin as time goes on, the collagen never disappears entirely, and scar tissue is never completely like normal skin.

When a skin graft is placed on the burn wound, the wound becomes smaller, and consequently there is less healing by contraction and the resulting abnormal scar is smaller. Scar tissue does form under the skin graft and around its edges, however, as the graft heals to the burn wound itself. Although the amount of scar tissue is reduced, scar tissue is present, as are *myofibroblasts*, specialized cells that cause contraction. Skin grafts do contract, and they frequently form tight scars. When skin grafts can be placed before five to seven days have passed after the injury, the resulting scarring is often diminished, possibly because myofibroblasts have not yet migrated into the wound.

Pathological burn scars

Formation of scar tissue is a normal part of healing. Some scars become pathological, however, and cause physical problems for the burn patient early on and even after the body has tried to remodel the scar tissue during the maturation phase of healing.

The most common pathological scar is the hypertrophic scar, which results from deep partial-thickness burns and full-thickness burns that have undergone the prolonged healing process (Figure 6.2). Hypertrophic scars are raised, red, and hard. They consist of thickened scar that is raised above the surface of the skin. They are usually firm or ropey to the touch, and they may be itchy or painful. Although these scars may widen, they stay within the bound of the original wound.

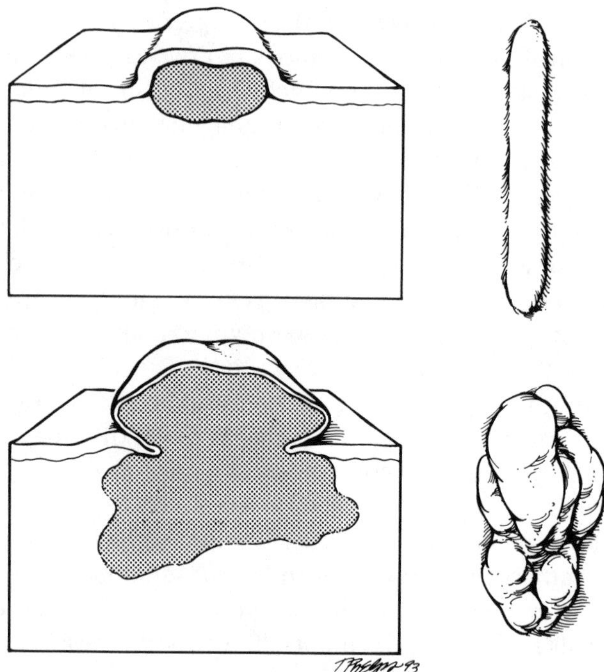

Figure 6.2. Excessive scarring which remains within bounds of the original wound is called a hypertrophic scar (*top*). Excessive scarring which extends beyond the bounds of the original wound is called a keloid (*bottom*).

Various means of applying pressure are used to compress areas of hypertrophic scarring as nonsurgical therapy (see Chapter 4). The application of pressure causes the collagen to lay down more normally within the scar and results in a softer, flatter scar. Compression garments and clear plastic face masks are used both to modify the development of hypertrophic scars and to treat them once they have developed (see Figure 4.6). Another nonsurgical therapy for small hypertrophic scars is injection of cortisone-type medications directly into the scar. These medications are thought to work by improving the ability of collagenase to break down scar tissue.

Keloids are similar to hypertrophic scars in appearance. The difference is that keloid scars grow beyond the bounds of the original wound (Figure 6.2). Their extensive growth makes keloid scars

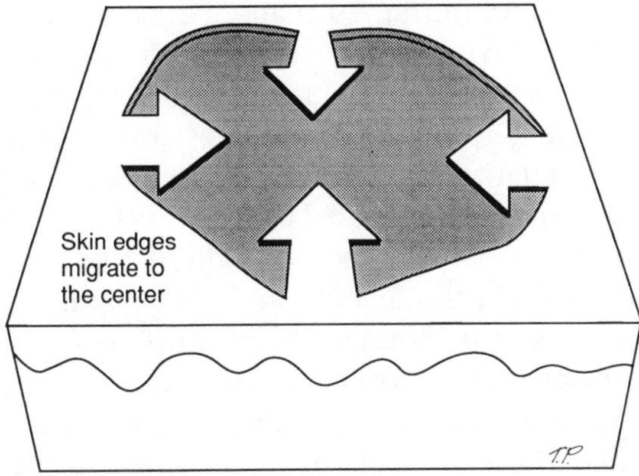

Figure 6.3. Contraction is the primary mode of wound healing for deep and full-thickness wounds.

innately more difficult to treat than hypertrophic scars. Nonoperatively, they are treated like hypertrophic scars. When they are removed surgically, keloid scars tend to return and to exceed the bounds of the surgical wound.

The third type of pathological scar occurs across a joint, limiting the movement of that joint (Figure 6.3). When the body responds to the loss of skin by contracting the wound, the contraction forces within the wound cause the skin on both sides of the joint to come together, and the distance across the joint is shortened. As a result, the joint may be pulled into an abnormal position, or it may not be possible for the person to completely extend the joint.

The scar tissue that develops across the joint is thick and rigid. It does not stretch. It can be improved somewhat by the application of pressure, splinting, and physical therapy. If these nonoperative treatments do not correct the problem, however, the surgeon will cut across the contracture and extend the joint. This surgery produces a new wound that is approximately the same size as the original burn injury (see Figure 6.9). A skin graft is placed onto this area, and if all goes well, the length of skin across the joint is restored along with full joint function.

Scars that remain an abnormal color for a long period of time are also considered pathological. Burn scars usually differ in color from normal skin early in the healing process and even long after the scar matures, frequently as long as 18 to 24 months after.

Gradually the color of the burn scar approximates the normal skin color, but it seldom completely matches the surrounding normal skin color. Dark-skinned individuals often have persistent *depigmentation*, resulting in patches of whiteness, or *hyperpigmentation*, resulting in extra-dark scars. Color inconsistencies that result from burn injury are most easily treated using corrective cosmetics (see Appendix B), with medical tattooing an alternative way of approximating normal skin color in small areas of depigmentation.

A final category of pathological scars consists of those that are inadequate in some way, most commonly scars that are thin and fragile, resulting in chronic reopening of the wound following minor trauma. These scars usually form when so much of the surrounding local tissue has been destroyed that contraction is insufficient to heal the wound. In this case, inadequate scar tissue forms and is covered with only a thin layer of epithelial cells. Correcting this problem usually requires cutting away the inadequate scar and covering the area with split-thickness skin grafts or flaps in its place (see below).

Pathological scars tend to develop within the first few months after healing and to improve with time. Hypertrophic scars and keloids will usually shrink and soften. Contractures will frequently lengthen and soften with time. Depigmented scars pigment (reacquire color) as long as 18 to 24 months after the initial burn injury. This tendency for scars to improve over time explains why there is an early emphasis on physical therapy and various modes of *nonsurgical* treatment of pathological scars.

The Timing and Techniques of Reconstructive Surgery

The waiting period

Unless scars pose an urgent functional problem or endanger a vital structure, reconstructive surgery for functional problems is deferred for 6 to 12 months, and reconstructive surgery for the correction of disfigurement is delayed as long as 12 to 18 months after burn injury. The delay sometimes eliminates the need for reconstructive surgery, or at least minimizes the extent of surgery required. Furthermore, surgery performed on a mature scar produces the best results, and the waiting period allows for scar maturation.

Undergoing reconstructive surgery before the end of the waiting period is fraught with dangers: complications can arise from the formation of excessive scar tissue after this surgery, for example, or the patient may become infected from bacteria in the hospital. In addition, the person will not be able to tolerate anesthesia or increased bleeding well at this point, because his or her general condition has been compromised metabolically and immunologically.

It is sometimes difficult for the burn survivor to be patient during this waiting period. But the wait will result in a better outcome, and the intervening time is not wasted. The period after discharge from the burn unit is a period in which recovery continues in the following ways: first, the person's metabolic and immunologic functions gradually return to normal and become stabilized after the wound has been closed; second, burn wounds continue to mature; and finally, the person gradually recovers physical, psychological, and social balance.

The burn survivor will be encouraged to keep busy during this period, possibly by returning to work (on a part-time basis if necessary) or by undertaking vocational rehabilitation, if necessary, to prepare for a new occupation. During this period, too, the burn survivor will begin to come to terms with the fact that his or her life has been changed and that, despite successful reconstructive surgery, many of the changes caused by the injury will be permanent. It takes different people different amounts of time to adapt to being a burn survivor. What many people discover, finally, is that not all of the changes brought by a burn injury are negative. Many burn survivors make very positive changes in their lives after suffering a severe burn injury.

During the waiting period the burn survivor will talk with experts in reconstructive surgery who will reassure the survivor while helping him to realize that rehabilitation will be a long and gradual process. The survivor and his family will have the chance to express concerns, both immediate and long-term, about the psychological and social effects of scarring, and they will be introduced to reconstructive procedures that will take place in the future. A definite plan for reconstructive surgery will be presented so that the burn survivor can look forward to continual improvement.

The importance of allowing burn scar maturation to take place before reconstructive surgery is performed cannot be overemphasized. The best course is to allow the pathological scars to be treated by the occupational therapist so that they become softer and paler before reconstructive surgery is performed. When burn scars are to be removed and replaced by other skin, it is best to allow a loose, mobile scar to develop over the underlying tissues before the scar is removed.

Definitions

Reconstructive surgery is the aspect of plastic surgery whose goal is correction of the dysfunction and disfigurement resulting from injury. Reconstructive surgery is surgery that deals with the repair or replacement of lost or damaged parts of the body.

Reconstructive surgery for burn injuries usually consists of replacing the skin lost or disfigured by the injury in order to correct the pathological scars described above. Deforming scars are cut out (excised), and the wound is either closed (if sufficient skin exists) or covered with new skin, a procedure called *resurfacing*. Also in reconstructive surgery, contractures are released (cut across), and skin is placed in the resulting wound after the joint is extended.

Reconstructive surgery differs from cosmetic surgery in that reconstructive surgery takes something that is abnormal and tries to make it as normal as possible, whereas *cosmetic surgery* takes something that is relatively normal, such as the effects of the aging process, and tries to make it better than normal.

The surgical correction of physical problems resulting from burns is a major component of the rehabilitation of the burn survivor. It is a difficult and lengthy process that may require numerous operations. Although the outcome of these operations will almost always fall short of the ideal, the reconstructive surgeon holds normal appearance as the ideal and strives to achieve it. Most operations are successful in terms of returning function, but the burn survivor can never be returned to completely normal function and appearance.

Grafts. As discussed in Chapter 1, a *graft* is tissue that is completely removed from the body, disconnected from its blood supply, and

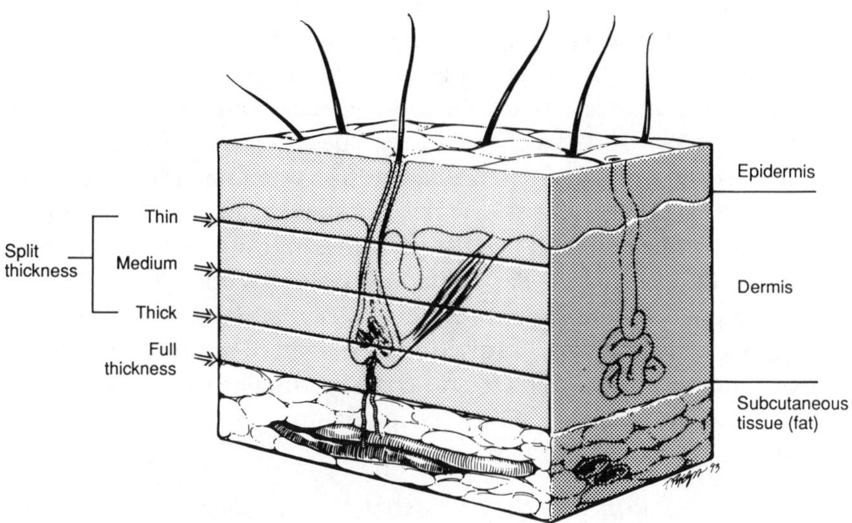

Figure 6.4. Normal skin, showing the thickness of different kinds of skin grafts.

replaced on a wound, where it lives by absorbing nutrients from the wound. The area from which tissue is taken to be donated to another area of the body is called the *donor site*. The *recipient site* is the wound that is in need of closure and which receives the tissue during reconstruction. Blood vessels from the wound generally grow into the graft within three or four days, resulting in the "take" of the graft.

Whereas most burn wounds that need to be closed by skin graft surgery are covered with split-thickness skin grafts during the acute burn recovery period, full-thickness grafts, composite grafts, and flaps are generally used for reconstructive surgery. When a *split-thickness graft* is taken, only a portion of the dermis is removed with the epidermis; a *full-thickness skin graft* involves removing the entire thickness of the skin for use as a graft (Figure 6.4).

Composite grafts contain more than one type of tissue, most commonly skin and cartilage from the ear, and are sometimes used to reconstruct facial features such as the nose, eyebrows, and upper lip. Split-thickness donor sites heal by epithelialization, but when a full-thickness or composite graft is taken, the donor site must be closed with sutures or, sometimes, with a split-thickness graft.

A *flap* is tissue that maintains its blood supply when moved to another area of the body. One advantage of flaps is that they do not contract, so secondary contracture can be avoided. A *local flap* is a flap that is moved to an area adjacent to its original donor site. A *distant flap* is a piece of tissue which is moved to an area that is not adjacent to the donor site. In the past, an extremity such as an arm was used to provide the flap from one area of the body to another. Today, however, the most common way of maintaining the blood supply to a distant flap is to disconnect the blood supply to the flap from the original donor site and connect the flap's blood vessels into blood vessels close to the recipient site using microvascular surgery. This is called a *free flap*.

Principles of reconstructive surgery

Before reconstructive surgery is undertaken, the deformity must be analyzed and the factors causing it must be diagnosed. The extent of reconstructive surgery is determined largely by how much skin has been destroyed by the burn. The skin deficit—the amount of missing skin—is often much greater than it seems, and therefore part of the surgeon's role is preparing the patient and those close to him for a substantial operation.

Restoration of function precedes reconstruction for appearance, with release of contractures the first priority, particularly contractures that endanger vital organs such as the eyes. Ideally, restoration of function and appearance can be achieved simultaneously, though this is not always possible. Surgeons do try to accomplish as many goals as possible during each operative procedure, however. This both minimizes the patient's exposure to anesthetics and reduces the overall length of the reconstructive period.

Scars can never be completely removed, but through plastic surgery they can be minimized, making them less noticeable. The techniques of reconstructive surgery are directed toward making scars smaller, thinner, and generally "better looking." In reconstructive surgery, burn scars are commonly moved so that they are hidden in the contours or *resting skin tension lines* (RSTL) of the face or the body (Figure 6.5). Scars lying within or parallel to the RSTL

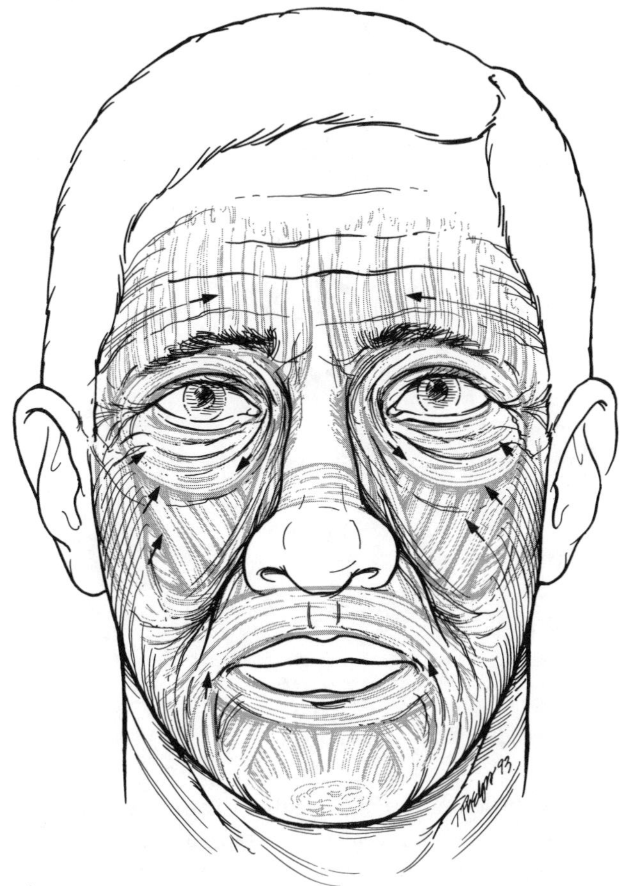

Figure 6.5. The resting skin tension lines, also called Langer's lines, lie perpendicular to the action of underlying muscles. Scars that run parallel to these lines are the least noticeable.

are generally better hidden than scars that run perpendicularly to the RSTL.

Local flaps are used whenever possible, because they provide the best color match, skin texture, and skin thickness for reconstruction. A *Z-plasty* is one of the most commonly used local flaps (Figure 6.6). With a Z-plasty, a long, straight line scar is broken into multiple broken lines. This makes the scar less visible and often

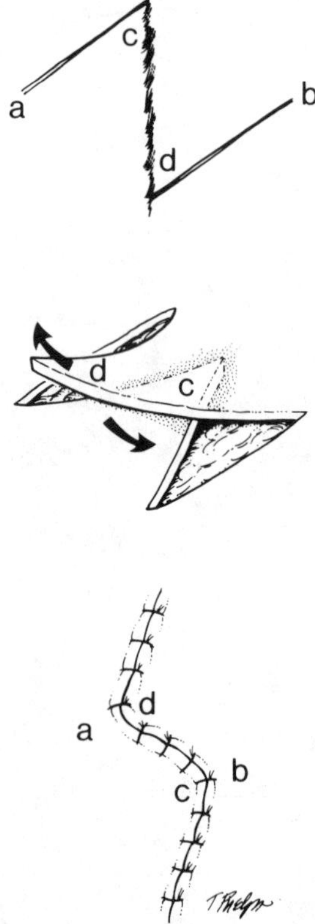

Figure 6.6. Z-Plasty breaks up and reorients the line of the scar and lengthens the scar. It is used to make the scar less noticeable and to release straight line contractures. This drawing shows how the scar will be lengthened and reoriented through surgery.

reorients the scar into the natural lines of the skin. Displaced anatomic structures can be restored to normal position with a Z-plasty, linear scars can be lengthened, and tension can be reduced along the length of the scar.

Another method of breaking a long scar into multiple broken lines is a W-plasty (Figure 6.7), which is performed in broad, open areas of skin where there is an excess of tissue, such as the cheek. The limbs of the resulting W are aligned better with the resting skin tension lines of the face than the original scar was, and the final scar is less noticeable.

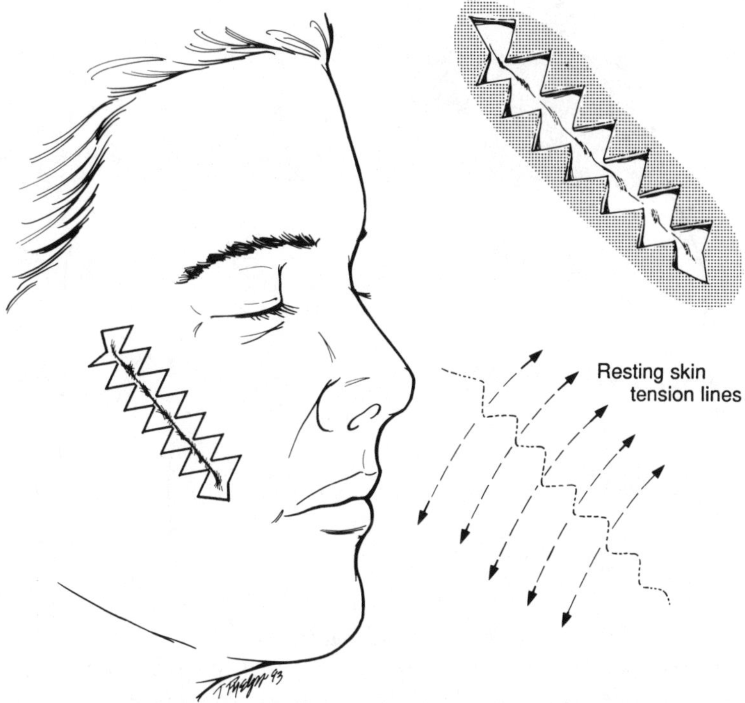

Figure 6.7. W-Plasty breaks up and reorients the line of the scar more nearly into resting skin tension lines. It is used to make the scar less noticeable. In this drawing, the existing scar and the outline for the W-plasty are shown on the face. The drawing in the upper right-hand corner shows the area of the skin that will be undermined; in this procedure, the edges of the W-plasty will be lifted in preparation for the surgery. The line shown at lower right shows what the healed new scar will look like; it will be oriented into the resting skin tension lines on the face.

A new technique for increasing the amount of local tissue available for flaps is *tissue expansion,* in which a deflated silicone balloon called a *tissue expander* is placed under normal skin next to the areas to be reconstructed (Figure 6.8). The balloon is inflated by injecting a saltwater solution into a valve on the balloon which can be felt through the skin. The inflation stretches the skin, and the body responds to this stretching by growing new skin. The procedure may be repeated several times—more saltwater being injected into the expander each time—until enough new skin is

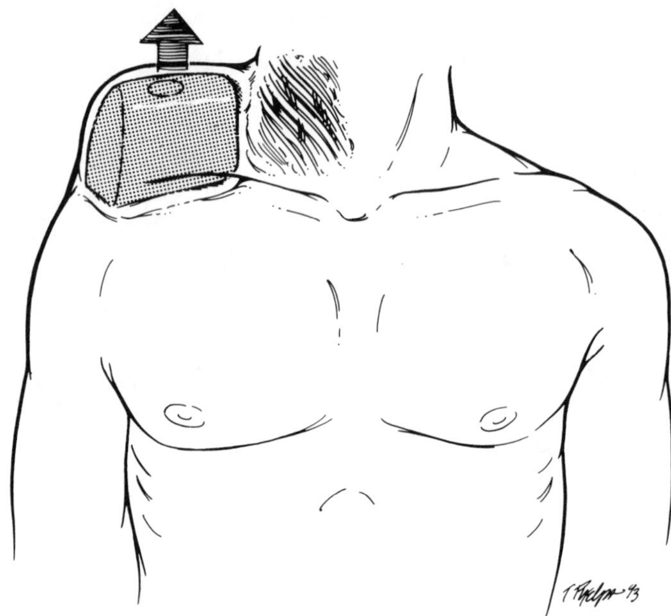

Figure 6.8. In tissue expansion, normal skin near the burn scar responds to stretching by growing more skin over the expander. In this drawing the tissue expander has been inserted under the skin on the shoulder, near the scar in the neck that will be grafted with the skin that grows during this procedure. A saltwater solution will be inserted into the valve, shown here on the top of the expander.

grown to reconstruct the adjacent defect after the tissue expander is removed.

When the areas of burn scarring are extensive, there may not be sufficient normal tissue to permit reconstruction by local flaps alone. In this case, full-thickness or thick split-thickness skin grafts are used to resurface large areas. These grafts also provide the best means of preserving fine facial features. Thick split-thickness skin is generally used for reconstructing the eyelid, for example, unless full-thickness eyelid skin is available from the eyelid on the opposite side. Color is best matched when local skin can be used as the donor site.

As a rule, the more dermis the graft contains, the less likely it is that the graft will change postoperatively. For most surgery performed to release contractures, full-thickness skin graft is the first choice, although the amount of full-thickness graft available often determines whether full-thickness or thick split-thickness grafts are used.

Distant flaps are used much less commonly for burn reconstruction. When a wound has neither adequate blood supply to support a skin graft nor adequate local flap tissue to provide full coverage, a distant flap reconstruction is used. A free muscle flap may be used to cover exposed skull where the overlying scalp has been destroyed, for example. Or hair-bearing skin flaps from the scalp may be used to reconstruct beard or eyebrows.

Throughout reconstruction, the medical staff will consider and nurture the well-being of the burn survivor as an individual. They will monitor the effects on the patient's emotional and social life of the original burn injury and of the reconstructive procedures. They will guide the patient in using such nonsurgical techniques of camouflaging scars as medical tattooing, corrective cosmetics, prostheses, and dermabrasion. They will follow up on the patient and monitor both splinting and proper fitting and wearing of compression garments to preserve the result of the reconstructive surgery. Follow-up is essential, and the patient and the medical team must work together to ensure that no aspect of follow-up is neglected.

Reconstructive Surgery on the Scalp and Face

The scalp

The most common scalp problem addressed by burn reconstruction surgery is the area of the burn scar called *burn alopecia* (*alopecia* means baldness), where hair and hair roots have been destroyed. Small areas of alopecia can be surgically removed and the resulting wound closed with stitches. Because scalp skin has a tough underlying layer (called *galea*), it does not stretch like skin in other areas of the body, and this limits the areas of scar that can be removed directly.

In the past, multiple scalp flap techniques were used to cover larger areas of alopecia, but tissue expansion is increasingly being used for reconstruction of scalp defects. With tissue expansion the hair-bearing scalp can be expanded, the scarred portion of the scalp excised, and the expanded hair-bearing scalp put in its place. No new hair is formed, but the space between hair follicles increases as the scalp expands, causing a thinning of the hair that is usually imperceptible.

Less common than alopecia in burn injury is complete loss of a portion or all of the scalp, with the result that the underlying skull is exposed. Because the skull bone has no blood supply on its surface to support a skin graft, a flap that has its own vascular system must be placed in this area. Usually a free muscle flap from a distant site is put in place, and a skin graft is placed on the muscle. This procedure is generally performed early in the course of recovery, to prevent infection of the skull bone. Once the skull has been covered in this way, the remaining defect can be treated like burn alopecia.

The face: aesthetic units

Burns of the face heal much like burns on other parts of the body, but the results of scarring can be much more devastating, because the face is constantly in view. The timing and technique of reconstructive surgery on the face are very important. Skin replacement of the face should be performed in aesthetic units; that is, grafts and flaps should be placed so that scars are located within naturally occurring lines of the face (for example, the lines around the nose and mouth) or lines of contour (the jaw line or the hairline).

Each of the areas of the face has specific requirements when it comes to reconstructive surgery.

The forehead is a surprisingly large expanse of skin, extending from the hairline to the eyebrows and from the outside corner of the eye back to the hairline above the ear. Although the natural skin lines of the forehead run horizontally, a vertical scar in the center of the forehead is often acceptable. Most small scars can be excised in a way that creates a horizontal scar and very little deformity. When the patient has large forehead scars, the forehead must be resurfaced, generally by placing a thick split-thickness graft as an aesthetic unit (with the scars in the hairline).

A hair-bearing full-thickness graft from the temple or behind the ear may yield an acceptable result for reconstruction of an *eyebrow*, but hair growth is usually sparse and unsatisfactory. The sparseness can be augmented using eyebrow pencil or by medical tattooing (which is permanent). Eyebrow prostheses are also available. Surgical transfer of small hair-bearing scalp flaps may be the procedure of choice.

To allow the upper *eyelids* to move freely, eyelid skin is very thin and delicate. Beneath the skin is the muscle, which helps to pump the film of tears over the eyeball and into the canals that drain tears into the nose. When scarring restricts the mobility of the eyelid, or when the eyeball is exposed when the eyelid is contracted, or pulled away, from the eyeball, the pumping action of the eyelid is compromised. Artificial lubricants are applied to protect the patient's corneas until reconstructive surgery can be performed. The eyes must be kept well lubricated, even if that means temporarily obscuring the patient's vision.

To reconstruct eyelids, full-thickness skin from the eyelid of the other eye is the ideal replacement for eyelid skin and is used if it is available. More often, thick split-thickness skin is used to release contractures of the eyelids (which are common following a burn injury involving the eyelid). The release of the eyelid will be overcorrected in surgery, and frequently this will make the eyelids appear large or droopy, but this overcompensation will correct itself in time, and the eyelids will appear more normal. Scars across the corners of the eyelid can restrict movement; they are corrected using Z-plasty flap techniques or skin graft.

False eyelashes or tattooed eyeliner can be used to substitute for the eyelashes.

Burn injury around the face and neck often results in partial or total *ear* loss. Ear reconstruction is often difficult because of burn scarring next to the ear. When nearby normal skin is available, this skin is used for reconstruction. Portions of the remaining ear can be used to reconstruct the general form of the ear. When the ear is totally missing, a vascularized deep tissue flap from under the scalp is used to cover a framework of rib cartilage, or sometimes plastic. This flap is subsequently covered with a skin graft. Prostheses that look very much like real ears are often the best solution when the entire ear is lost.

As with the ear, reconstruction of the *nose* is difficult. Patients whose faces have been burned often have retracted nostrils, so that some of the nasal lining is turned out rather than in. Reconstruction involves releasing the scar contracture, making up the tissue deficit caused by the burn, replacing the nasal lining in its anatomic location, and resurfacing the nose with local flaps, full-thickness grafts, or, sometimes, a composite graft of skin and cartilage. When the nose is missing, skin from the forehead or from other areas of the body is placed over a cartilage framework to shape a new nose. Nasal prostheses are also available.

The *mouth,* like the eyelid, is a dynamic structure whose mobility can be affected by burn scar contractures. Small linear contractures can be released by Z-plasty technique. When large portions of the upper or lower lip are scarred, these areas must be replaced by skin graft applied as an aesthetic unit. Technically, the area around the mouth consists of five aesthetic units. The upper lip consists of the dimple in the middle of the lip flanked by two lateral aesthetic units extending out to the nasolabial crease (the groove between the nose and the corners of the month). The lower lip is an inverted U-shaped aesthetic unit surrounding the prominence of the chin itself, which is the fifth aesthetic unit. The contour of the dimple in the upper lip can be duplicated by using a composite graft of ear skin and cartilage.

Scarring often occurs in the corner of the mouth, restricting the mouth's ability to open. These scars can occur when the face is burned or when the mouth is specifically burned, usually when a child bites into an electrical cord, receiving an electrical arc burn in this area. The shortening and rounding of the corner of the mouth is usually corrected by releasing the scar contracture. The resulting wound is covered with a flap of tissue from one of the lips to the other lip wound, followed by coverage of the donor lip defect with mucous membrane from inside the mouth.

Cheeks are another large aesthetic unit of the face. When the cheeks are scarred, the skin may be discolored and the person may lose facial expression (as a result of tight or firm scars). Contour deformities may be present from hypertrophic scars that are difficult to cover with cosmetics.

Hyperpigmentation can sometimes be permanently improved with skin bleaching agents or chemical peels, although cosmetics usually are adequate to camouflage the discoloration of burn scars. Corrective cosmetics now exist which remain in place in water and when the skin comes in contact with clothing and people.

When tightness occurs as a result of contractures, and when

large areas of hypertrophic scarring are present, the cheek is often resurfaced using a full-thickness skin graft or a flap of skin from the neck or shoulder. The aesthetic unit of the cheek is so large that a tissue expander may be used to expand the donor tissue so that it will cover the entire cheek unit.

Small hypertrophic scars and contractures can be corrected or improved through excision of the scars and subsequent closure with Z-plasty or W-plasty.

Reconstructive Surgery on the Body: Joint Contractures

Burn scar contractures can develop across any of the major joints of the body, though they are most common in the neck, across the shoulder joint or armpit area (axilla), and on the hands, wrists, elbows, knees, and feet. Contractures often severely limit function of the related body part. Early burn physical therapy strives to prevent these contractures as much as possible and to modify the scar tissue to correct or improve contractures if they form. If the contractures are significant between 6 and 12 months after the burn, however, reconstructive surgery is performed to release the contractures (Figure 6.9).

Because *neck* extension is necessary to place a breathing tube easily (and the anesthesiologist must place a breathing tube down the neck during surgical procedures), release of a neck contracture is often the first reconstructive operation performed on a severely burned person. The neck is less important aesthetically than the face, because it is relatively well hidden and can be further hidden with clothing. But the function of the neck is extremely important: the neck allows the head to move. Each of the seven vertebrae (spinal bones) that make up the spine in the neck is separated by a joint that allows the head to move over a very wide range. Scar contractures restrict the movement of these joints, most commonly when a contracture lies across the front of the neck and restricts the extension of the neck.

A neck contracture is most frequently released through a simple incision and skin grafting that allows the neck to extend, although Z-plasties and other local flap techniques are also used. The skin graft is placed over the resulting wound, with the size of the graft

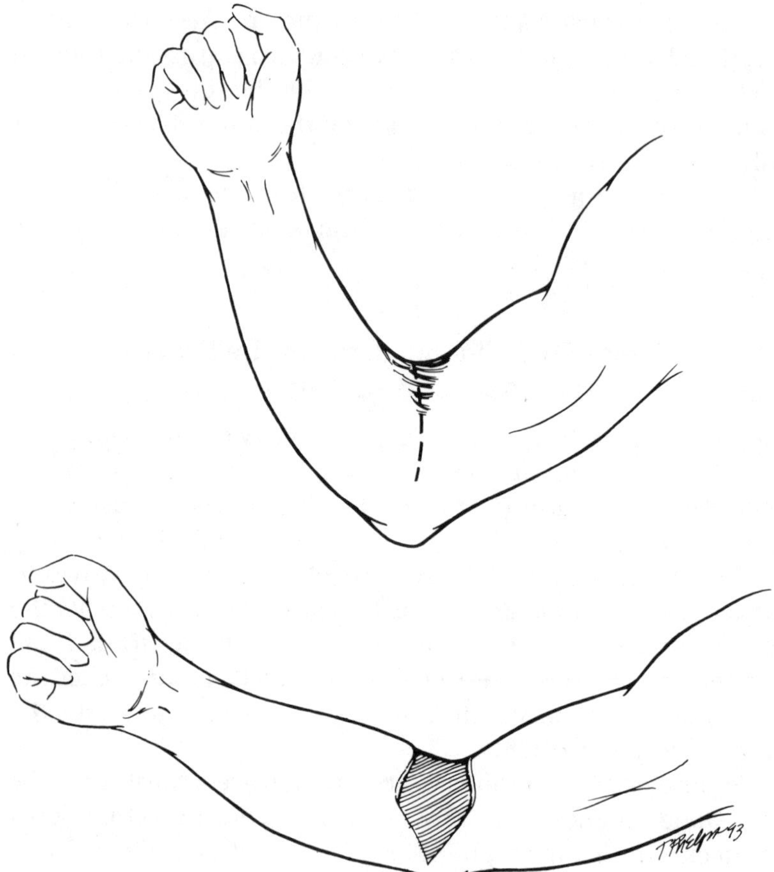

Figure 6.9. When an elbow contracture release is performed, an incision is made across the contracture. This opens into a wound that illustrates a loss of tissue when the elbow is extended. The wound is grafted with full-thickness skin.

usually being quite large. Grafts generally take well in the neck tissues, with the exception of grafts over the larynx (the "Adam's apple"), the movement of which interferes with the healing of the graft.

Small contracture scars in the neck can be excised along the resting skin tension lines. Scars that run against the RSTL are often reoriented toward the RSTL using local flap surgery.

Tracheostomy scars can be disfiguring, since they are often wider and depressed relative to the surface of the skin. When they are attached to the underlying larynx, as sometimes occurs, tracheostomy scars move in an unsightly way when the person swallows. The appearance of tracheostomy scars can be improved through reconstructive surgery.

Reconstructive surgery on the *hand* addresses the problems that remain despite intensive physical and occupational therapy, which begins early in the course of burn treatment. The functions of the hand result from the complex interactions of the various components of the hand. Loose skin on the back of the hand and sensitive, thicker skin on the palm cover the tendons, ligaments, nerves, muscles, bones, and joints. Contractures of these many joints and loss of skin sensitivity can interfere with the interactions that allow the hand to function as a fine instrument. These problems must be addressed.

Burn scars on the hand often result in stiffness and limited motion. Even when the burn seems to involve only the skin, the restriction of hand function can be severe. Contractures of the fingers are released using grafts and flaps, and sometimes the ligaments around the joints must be released as well, in a surgical procedure called a *capsulectomy*, in which a portion of the joint capsule is removed.

As noted earlier in this book, deep burns of the hands can expose tendons and nerves, frequently resulting in the amputation of a finger or fingers. Amputations can sometimes be performed in such a way as to minimize the appearance of the loss of a finger.

The most common effect of burn scars on the *feet* is contracture of the dorsum (the top or back) of the foot, which causes the toes to be pulled back. A person whose toes are hyperextended (pulled back) is forced to put all of his weight on the balls of his feet when walking, resulting in an unnatural gait. When a child's feet have been burned (most frequently in scald injuries from bathing or spillage of hot liquids), the growth of the foot may be disturbed.

Contractures of the feet are released as soon as it becomes apparent that therapy and splinting alone will not correct the problem. Release and grafting usually correct the contracture and the hyperextension of the toes, leaving webbing between the toes. The webbing rarely interferes with function and can be left in place until the child is much older and desires reconstructive surgery for its removal.

Scar contractures on the *trunk* can interfere with movement, particularly if a tight scar is the continuation of a scar contracture across a joint such as in the neck or shoulders. These contractures are also released using grafts or local flaps.

When hypertrophic scarring develops over the large areas of the chest, back, and abdomen, resurfacing is not possible, since it would require too large a skin graft and would result in disfigurement of the skin graft donor site. Also, the split-thickness skin graft that would be used is subject to recurrent contracture and color changes, and so it would likely recreate the very problems it was intended to correct.

The development of techniques for the grafting of skin grown in tissue culture may eventually make it possible for reconstructive surgeons to resurface large areas of pathological scars without having to take split-thickness grafts from large donor sites. Cultured skin (*cultured epidermal autografts*, or CEA) is already being used in the treatment of severely burned patients. Not only has this technique saved lives, it has shown promise for use in reconstructive surgery, since the areas grafted with CEA show less tendency toward hypertrophic scarring than areas grafted with tissue from donor sites. Currently research is also under way to synthesize dermis. In the future, then, reconstructive surgeons may be able to use these components from outside the body to restore the body's function and form.

The physical dysfunction and deformity resulting from a major burn injury is almost always seen initially as an overwhelming burden to those who have the misfortune to experience it. But almost always, too, emotional and spiritual healing takes place along with physical reconstruction and physical healing. The human spirit, after a period of mourning what has been lost, overcomes and adapts to even the most difficult of circumstances. With the help of family, friends, and the rehabilitation team, burn survivors recover their health and shine through their scars.

Part III

Looking to the Future

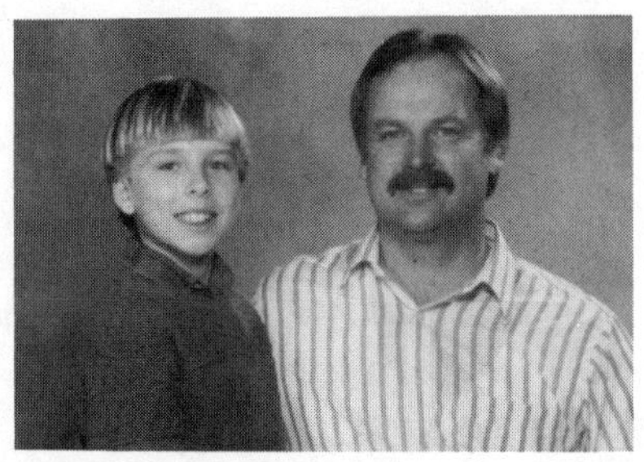

I knew something was wrong when I got up Thanksgiving morning and Mom was gone. We had just talked the night before about making the pumpkin pies to take to MiMi's and Pap's for dinner. Pumpkin pies were Mom's and my specialty. We had gone to the orchard and picked out the perfect pumpkin. I knew Mom wouldn't have gone away on the day we were making pies unless something was wrong.

Another thing. Our neighbor was sitting at our kitchen table drinking coffee and looking real serious. He had never babysat for me before. I didn't want him to think I was a scared baby—after all, I was six years old and in the first grade—so I said I was crying because I was sick. He had just started to hunt for Tylenol when the phone rang. It was Mom. She told me that Dad had been in an accident. I thought she meant a car accident. She said that Aunt Lynn and Uncle Gary would be up soon to get me and that she would see me later. It helped to know that Mom was okay, but I was scared about Dad. Dad and I were buddies. We did lots of things together. I helped him to farm and work on the house, and he played ball with me and helped me with my flash cards. I didn't want my Dad to be hurt bad.

My aunt and uncle came and our neighbor went home. My aunt started to wash and pack my clothes. She had tears in her eyes, but I didn't ask any questions. I wanted to talk to my Mom. When Mom, my other uncle, and Gran came, Mom sat real close to me on the sofa and held me tight. She said that there had been an accident at the aluminum plant where my Dad worked and that he had been burned. She said that she was going to Baltimore to be near Dad's hospital and that Gran would be staying with me. She said we had to be brave and help Dad to get well. I was very scared, but I didn't cry—I just held real tight to Mom.

We ate Thanksgiving dinner at Gran's. MiMi had cooked the turkey and made the pumpkin pie. Then Mom left for Baltimore, and I started the long, lonely wait for my Dad to come home.

The next day, Gran and I started something that we did almost every day until Dad came home. We went to the card shop and I picked out the get-well cards to send to Dad. We got lots of cards with funny animals on them. Every day, we wrote Dad a note on the card and we tried hard to be funny. We told Dad about school and about the snowman that Gran helped me make when it snowed. It was not a very good snowman. Even the dog thought it was pretty bad—he peed on it. Mom said Dad really laughed when he got that card. It felt good to know I made Dad laugh. Somehow that made him feel a little closer to me. Sometimes I made Dad presents and put them in the cards. One day I sent him a paper crown.

When I went back to school on Monday, I took the article from the newspaper that told about my Dad's accident. I also took the melted aluminum Dad had once given me, to help the kids understand how my Dad got hurt. Everybody was real nice to me, and all the kids in my class made cards to send to Dad.

The phone rang all the time after Dad was hurt. I didn't know how bad he was hurt, so I listened to everything Gran said on the phone. Sometimes I would sneak upstairs and listen in on the extension, but Gran caught me. She asked me if I wanted to know anything. I was really scared my Dad would die, but I was afraid to ask that. I was afraid it would come true.

Mom called every night to tell us how Dad was. I told her that I wanted to see my Dad, but she said kids couldn't come to the hospital. She said that kids have lots of germs from school and that Dad could get an infection from those germs. I thought maybe she just didn't want me to see Dad hurt so bad. She told me that she read my cards to Dad every day and that she put the pictures I sent on his bulletin board. That night, I couldn't sleep. I was afraid that my Dad couldn't see. When I asked Gran, she said that he could see. She said his face wasn't burned. I hoped everybody was telling the truth.

The next day Mom bought a camera that makes a picture right away. She sent pictures of Dad so I could see that his face was all right. That really helped. He was wearing the crown I had sent him, and he didn't look sick at all. He had a lot of bars that looked like a jungle gym over his bed to help him move around. His legs were all covered up and he had bandages on his arms, but he looked just like my Dad always looked and he looked great to me.

The doctors did a really funny thing to my Dad. They grew his skin.

Mom said they took a little piece of Dad's skin and flew it to Boston. Then they put it in a dish with some special stuff and it grew. When it was ready, they flew the new skin back and the doctors fastened it to Dad's legs and arm. Mom says they call that cultured skin and that it even had its own seat on the plane. Its ticket said "Epi Dermis." Mom came home once a week while Dad was in the hospital. She brought me surprises that Dad sent me. Little packages of strawberry jam from Dad's tray were my favorite. She brought pictures of my Dad and his room. He had all of my cards on his bulletin board. I sure wished I could see my Dad and hug him.

The second week in December, the phone rang one evening and it was my Dad! He said he told the nurse to wheel his bed out to the phone because he had to talk to his boy. He sounded wonderful. He told me that he loved me and that he was going to get well and come home. I knew that was the truth because my Dad doesn't lie to me. I didn't have any trouble going to sleep that night.

Gran and I went Christmas shopping for Mom and Dad. I got Mom some dish towels and Dad a pair of sweat pants because he wouldn't be able to wear regular pants for a long time. At the Christmas shop at school, I got Mom beads and Dad funny cards. MiMi and Pap and I got a live Christmas tree in a pot. MiMi and I strung popcorn and cranberries and hung them on the tree. I put Mom and Dad's presents under the tree and mine, too. I wanted to wait until Dad came home to open the presents with him.

A week before Christmas, MiMi and Pap took me to the hospital to see my Dad. He was in a funny bed that had a top like a chair. His legs were all covered up and we had to be very careful not to hurt them. Mom wheeled him out to the lounge and we played games and colored and hugged and hugged.

Mom said I couldn't come to visit Dad on Christmas because he was going to have grafting that week. That means they took the good skin off of Dad's belly and fastened it to his hurt legs. So Mom came home to Gran's for Christmas dinner and then took Dad's dinner back to him. The people where Dad and Mom worked sent Santa Claus to bring me lots of presents. I saved them all until Dad could come home. Everybody tried to be merry, but it was a sad, lonely Christmas without my Dad.

The first day of January, Gran and I put up a new calendar. Every day we put a sticker on it to count off the days until Dad could come home. I was really starting to get excited. Gran said I could stay home from school when Dad came home. Finally, the day came. We blew up balloons and MiMi brought a "Welcome Home" banner to put over the door. We waited and waited. About three o'clock, Mom pulled the station wagon in the driveway and my Dad got out of the back seat very slowly. He looked tired, but my Dad walked into our house on January 20. Almost three months after he was burned, my Dad was home!

My Dad's legs looked real bad when he came home. They had to be washed and bandaged every morning. They were just like two big pieces of meat and blood ran from them and dripped on the floor when he walked. I was real scared at first, but Mom taught me how to help. I got real good running to get gauze and salve and Ace bandages. It took Mom, the nurse, and me an hour and a half to get Dad's legs fixed in the morning. One good thing though, they didn't hurt, and slowly they started to heal.

A week after Dad came home, we had Christmas at our house. All our family came. We had turkey and trimmings and opened our presents. Everybody talked about miracles and that God had answered our prayers. I knew that was true because Gran and I had prayed hard for Dad to get well and come home. We all laughed and hugged and ate a lot. That day really felt like Christmas.

At first, Dad had to go back to the hospital every week, but as he got better, he only had to go once a month. After Dad was home for a while, he started physical therapy three times a week. I went with Dad a couple of times. They have all these neat machines that stretch muscles so that they can get stronger and don't shrink. Dad went in a cab because he couldn't drive. Now he drives himself. The people at the hospital made my Dad a rubber suit. He has to wear it all the time. It looks like brown long underwear. It's called a "Jobst."

My Dad is real famous. The newspaper reporter did an article on my Dad, and it was on the front page of the paper. He was also on TV when he came home from the hospital. I loved it. I told everybody. I'm proud of my Dad and so glad he is home.

Every day my Dad gets a little better. His legs still aren't healed all the way, but he bandages them himself in the morning. It's a piece of cake now. The nurse only comes once a week. He can walk without the walker. The doctor says he will need to be operated on to straighten his knees, but I'm not scared. I know my Dad will be all right. The newspaper reporter said I was a brick when Dad was in the hospital. I know I get that from my Dad.

People say that our lives will never be the same. I guess that's true. After all, I'm seven now and I have a dog and a little brother named Scott. My Dad can't do all the things he used to do, but I'm getting bigger every day. Maybe he won't ever be able to play ball with Scott like he did with me, but that's okay, I'm Scott's big brother and I'll play ball with him and Dad can just keep on being our wonderful, wonderful Dad.

Bryan Haines

Chapter 7

Organized Support

A burn injury places a great deal of physical and psychological stress on the burn survivor and his or her family. As discussed earlier in this book, the staff social worker, counselor, psychologist, and psychiatrist help to identify and manage any psychological and social problems that develop as a result of burn trauma. In fact, the personal and professional traits of *all* the members of the burn team create and color the relationships that develop between the medical team and patients and patients' families and friends. Special relationships often develop in the burn unit, and lifelong friendships are formed. These relationships can play a significant role in the lives of everyone involved.

Organized support services offer an additional, and essential, resource for those affected by a burn injury. Some people do in fact respond more positively to support offered in an informal setting than they do to more formal, clinical services. The purpose of this chapter is to describe the kinds of organized support which are available to burn survivors and to their loved ones beyond the clinical setting.

Survivor Groups

Local

An adult burn survivor group provides the opportunity for a burn survivor to meet other burn survivors. Such a group can help the person avoid feeling isolated; it can also be helpful and reassuring for the burn survivor to meet others who have had experiences similar to his own. A burn survivor group is designed to help facilitate the person's adjustment to the sometimes devastating consequences of a burn injury.

The group can be organized in any number of ways, but a self-motivated group that receives encouragement from a group coordinator is usually very effective. Anyone who has been treated at a burn facility, anyone who continues to receive outpatient services, and anyone who is currently a patient in the hospital can benefit from participating in group discussions or from simply listening to others.

Individuals are invited and encouraged to attend the group as soon as they are able to get out of bed. Such early involvement introduces burn survivors to an invaluable support system that can help them cope with their hospitalization, the rehabilitation program, and their return home. New members of the group who are still wrapped in bandages and are confined to a wheelchair are reassured and inspired by other people in the group who have recovered after sustaining a similar burn injury. The members of survivor groups find this support invaluable. In fact, one member said that just seeing people who were burned and made it back to life really helped him.

Members informally and openly discuss issues of concern to themselves as well as more general issues of mutual concern. One person may talk about his frustrations with being a patient in the burn unit, including the lack of privacy, the intrusions at all times of the day and night, and the dependence on others to feed him and put him on the bedpan. Another person may complain about the pain of therapy and the discomfort of wearing pressure garments and splints. Someone may share her concern over an upcoming surgery and the scarring that will result; other people in the group may respond by showing her their skin grafts and donor sites.

Anxieties about returning home and about family relationships and household responsibilities are often discussed. People also worry about what they will and will not be able to do in the future. One man told the group that he would need as much help as his two-year-old just to get up, get dressed, and eat breakfast. "What will my wife think of me?" he asked. "Will she see me as a husband or as another child?"

Someone who was injured at work may talk about being worried about returning to the scene of the accident and working there again. Someone who will not be able to return to work may talk about how much he will miss it and what he can do to occupy his time instead.

For people who have visible scars, reentering society can be especially difficult. "It wasn't until I tried to return to a somewhat normal life that I discovered that society felt that facial scars and an abnormal appearance are very distinct disabilities. Everywhere I went, people would stare; they would often nudge their friends and point me out. Sometimes people would ask me rude questions." Venting anger and embarrassment in a supportive setting can provide a welcome relief. People in the group can also provide suggestions about and rehearse how to respond to stares and questions. This helps prepare people to feel more comfortable in public settings.

One person related that after he returned home, his family and friends seemed uncomfortable around him. "My family wouldn't talk about what happened to me or how they were feeling about it. My friends would call and promise to visit but never come." Someone else in the group told a similar story about an old friend who turned away from her in a grocery store. It helped for members of the group to reassure one another that this was a common experience and that it involved a reaction to the physical appearance of burn scars but had nothing to do with the personality or style of the burn survivor.

Within a safe group environment, burn survivors have the opportunity to share their burn-related experiences and to offer support and encouragement to one another. This type of support is often more effective than the reassurances of family members and health professionals. As one burn survivor stated, "Anyone can tell you that they understand how you feel, but only someone else who has been burned can mean it."

A variety of group social activities may be organized to encourage reintegration into society and to foster friendships. Such activities include holiday parties, picnics, sporting events, games, educational and motivational conferences, and community outreach projects. Burn center staff are often included in these activities, which then serve as a reunion of sorts. Members of the group often develop networks of support which can be highly valuable outside the group setting. Knowing that a supportive, understanding person is just a phone call away can provide invaluable reassurance during difficult times.

A visitation program is often incorporated into an adult burn survivor support group. In such a program, members of the group meet individually with hospital inpatients who are not able to or who are not ready to attend the group meetings. Burn survivor visitors can answer questions and provide encouragement as no one else can. The focus of these visits varies according to the patient's needs. Visits may consist of casual and friendly conversation or of light recreation (such as a card game), or they may consist of sharing personal experiences and stories about adjusting to a burn injury. Family members and friends may also benefit from such visits.

A pediatric or child burn survivor support group is a valuable support service, giving young burn survivors an opportunity to help one another and themselves and have fun at the same time. Within such a group, a child can share feelings and recount hospital experiences while meeting and socializing with other children who have been burned. In this setting, children are given the chance to voice their opinions and concerns to a peer group whose members will listen to them and care about them. They can talk about their physical and emotional pain to other children who will fully understand their feelings.

In the child burn survivor group, time is often spent discussing the reaction of other children to the child's burn scars and altered appearance. Children can be cruel: they often tease each other and call each other names. The burn survivor will probably be on the receiving end of some of this cruelty. One girl with facial burn scars quietly told the group about the kids at school, who called her "fried chicken." This prompted other children to add up the long list of names they have been called by other children. Although it is difficult for adults to offer an explanation for this name-calling, the group leader can tell the group that children often behave that way when someone looks different. The group leader and children in the group readily offer suggestions for dealing with the situation. "I just say that I was burned and walk away," one boy said. "Even though I look different now, I'm the same person I was before."

Within the group setting, young burn survivors do not feel

different. They feel special. They can safely share their stories and develop friendships that will strengthen their self-esteem and confidence.

The social worker at your hospital can put you in contact with survivor organizations in your area, or you can contact any of the burn care facilities listed in Appendix C.

National

Within the last few years the idea of organized support has spread. Currently, there are three national burn organizations in the United States: the American Burn Association, the Phoenix Society, and the National Burn Victim Foundation. Each organization offers a variety of services. For example, the American Burn Association, the parent organization of professionals engaged in burn treatment, research, teaching, and rehabilitation, sponsors a number of special interest groups that meet during the Burn Association's annual national meeting. One such group is the Burn Survivor Group.

Although these larger and more formally organized groups are less intimate than the small, local survivor groups, they fulfill an important role: that of national advocacy. Injury in general and burn injury in particular are tremendously underfunded at the federal level when compared with diseases such as AIDS, cancer, and high blood pressure, so there is a great deal to be said for national visibility.

If you would like additional information, contact the American Burn Association at 800-548-2876. The Phoenix Society is located at 11 Rust Hill Road, Levittown, Pennsylvania 19056. Burn survivors and their families may call the Phoenix Society toll free at 800-888-BURN; others can reach the society by calling 215-946-BURN. The National Burn Victim Foundation is located at 32–34 Scottland Road, Orange, New Jersey 07050. The foundation can be reached by calling 201-676-7700.

Family Support Groups

A family support group is composed of spouses, significant others, siblings, and close friends of the burn survivor. The purpose of the group is to provide an opportunity for family members and friends to express their feelings and discuss the impact of the trauma on their lives.

While the burn survivor carries physical, often visible signs of injury, family and friends do not, and their special needs are often overlooked. The family may have difficulty coping with the long hours spent at the hospital, the numerous demands placed on them, and the unexpected intrusion of trauma into their lives, and because of their concern for the burn survivor, they may not recognize their own need for support and assistance.

A family support group can deal with such issues by providing a safe, nurturing, nonjudgmental environment in which group members can express their fears and their feelings of helplessness, anger, and guilt. Group members benefit not only from sharing their own emotions but also from listening to others express similar feelings, and from learning how other people have coped in a situation that is similar to theirs.

Just as children often befriend each other while in the hospital, members of families may also form friendships during the long hours spent at the hospital. Waiting rooms often serve as informal support settings as families share concern for their injured members. One mother encouraged another mother to go home and rest, assuring her that she would keep an eye on her child, too.

Members of a family support group often direct the group themselves by raising issues and concerns they wish to explore, or a group facilitator may take an active role by introducing topics (for example, intimacy, sexuality, or guilt) that otherwise may not be mentioned. Generally, an informal, round-table discussion allowing for participation by each member is successful.

Camps

Beneficial to many young burn survivors is a camp designed especially for them. Since their inception, burn camps have spread rapidly around the world. The primary emphasis of camp is to increase the camper's self-esteem by establishing positive relationships with peers who have had similar experiences (Figure 7.1). At camp, recreational, educational, and therapeutic activities combine to create an enjoyable experience for the campers.

Many burn camps offer a week-long, residential setting and a

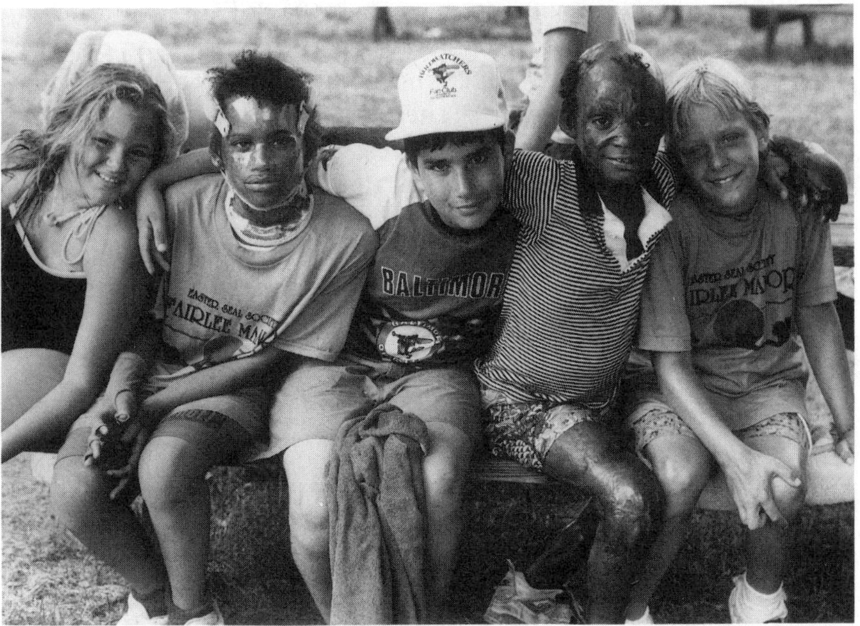

Figure 7.1. Happy campers

variety of outdoor activities including swimming, canoeing, horseback riding, arts and crafts, nature appreciation, and sports. These activities encourage young burn survivors to try things that they may have done before their injury but not since, and to simply experience new and challenging activities. Many camps also include a variety of burn-specific activities, conducted under the supervision of staff members knowledgeable in pediatric burn care, to provide campers with the opportunity to explore issues related to their injuries and others that may be important to them.

Frequently an adult burn survivor is invited to visit the camp and share his or her story with the children. After telling the children what happened, what problems he has as a result, and how he deals with them, the adult encourages the children to share their own stories. He then guides the conversation so that a variety of challenging issues are addressed, including how it feels to be burned or to be seen as different by other people, how the children feel about their scars, and what it's like to be teased and called names.

Another camp activity that encourages the child to explore how she feels about herself is body drawing. The child lies on a large piece of paper, and the outline of her body is traced. Then the child is asked to color in the outline. The result is often interesting: some children include their scars, pressure garments, and splints, while others do not. When the drawing is finished, the child is asked to explain it to the group. Group members then ask the child questions to help her identify what she sees as positive and negative qualities about herself, and to provide support and peer acceptance.

All young burn survivors are candidates for camp, although different camps have different requirements in terms of age and physical abilities. Families usually are not required to pay to send a child to camp, since most camps are funded by hospital affiliations, private donations, and grants. The social worker or psychologist at your regional burn center (see Appendix C) can provide you with information about the camps in your area. Or you can contact the American Burn Association and ask to speak to someone in the Burn Camp Special Interest Group.

School Programs

An important step along the road to recovery for children and adolescent burn survivors occurs when they return to school. The burn survivor should return to his or her normal school environment as soon as wound healing and physical condition permit. While early school reentry is beneficial to both the child and his or her classmates in the long run, the actual event is often a time of anxiety and concern for the child, the family, and school alike. This transition can be made easier with the help of a school reentry team.

A reentry team is composed of burn center staff members with experience in the acute and long-term care of pediatric and adolescent burn patients. Frequently these team members have worked with the returning child during his or her hospital stay and are familiar with the child's individual needs.

Before the child returns to school, a member of the team obtains the family's consent to contact the child's school to arrange the visit. The team also contacts the child's teacher to learn more about the child's learning style and how the child related to classmates prior to injury. This information helps the team prepare a personalized visit to best meet the unique needs of each child in the class.

On the day of the visit, the returning child may or may not be present. This decision is made by the child and his or her parents. (*Parents* are strongly advised to attend the reentry program, however.) If the child is reluctant to attend the reentry program because he is nervous or fearful of rejection or ridicule, he should not be forced to attend. After the presentation, the parents and the team members should reassure the child that the class accepted the news of the injury and were understanding and eager to help in any way possible. Perhaps the child would like to meet with a few teachers and close friends after the visit.

If the child is comfortable with the idea of participating, her participation ought to be encouraged. Often the child enjoys the special attention of the class and will benefit from telling the class directly about her experience and answering their questions. Team members take special care to make the child and her classmates comfortable.

The program usually begins with the introduction of the team members and a discussion of their roles in the burn center. Basic information about burn injuries and some specifics of treatment are presented. If the child is in active rehabilitation, the importance of exercise and the use of splints are reviewed. There is a careful discussion of scarring and the wearing of compression garments. Time is spent dealing with the feelings and fears of both the burned child and his or her classmates. Burn prevention basics are reviewed. Finally, there is a question and answer period.

A visit to the school by the burn team is geared to the ages and abilities of the children attending. The program can be adapted for all ages, from preschool to high school and even for children with special needs. Many teaching techniques are employed in the program. Team members may dress as they would in the burn unit, in hat, gown, and mask; students may try on dressings, splints, and compression garments. And demonstrations involving puppets and dolls or audiovisual materials like slides may be presented. Students in all age groups are encouraged to interact with the team members and to ask questions.

There is no limit to the questions asked by children during a class visit, and the questions range from the simple to the complex: How does it feel to be burned? Will it hurt if I touch his burn scar? Can she play games with us? Will the scars ever go away? What happens in the operating room? The students are given freedom to ask any question they may have; no question is too silly or dumb. The team also talks with the students about the fears of the burned child as well as the fears of his classmates.

After the reentry visit, team members try to maintain contact with the school so that the burn survivor's progress can be monitored and additional intervention can be provided if necessary.

Volunteer and Business Activities

Many burn survivors build a tremendous amount of self-esteem and obtain notable satisfaction by volunteering for various activities associated with burn units or burn services. Success stories abound, but perhaps the best known is that of the severely burned firefighter who, after recovering, returned to active duty in his fire department. No longer able to fight fires, he became the public relations officer and was eventually elevated to national office with the international union of firefighters, where for many years he performed invaluable service by promoting the cause of survivors of fire.

Other burn survivors work with recovered patients as teachers, therapists, fund raisers, cosmetologists; several have even started businesses, providing products and supplies that serve the special needs of burn survivors. We know of one young survivor who because of his burn experience changed his academic program from liberal arts and teaching to premedical study. So strong was his motivation to help others that he became a doctor.

Church Groups

Church groups are among the best-organized and strongest groups in providing emotional and physical support to their members and their families. If a burn patient or his or her family belongs to a church, even if they have not been very active members in the past, they may find a great deal of satisfaction and solace in calling upon a church group for help in this time of distress. For individuals who do not belong to a church and do not have a pastor but wish to obtain counseling and help from a member of the clergy, the hospital chaplain is available at all times.

Organized support services are a valuable source of assistance for burn survivors both during hospitalization and after the return home. By sharing experiences and positive coping strategies, burn survivors can help one another through rehabilitation and the return to everyday life.

There is no reason to go through this difficult time alone. We encourage you to ask your hospital or one of the national support organizations for information about support services.

Chapter 8

Prevention: Spread the Word

You may think this chapter is the last thing you want to read: you have a loved one in the hospital or you are a burn victim yourself, and what you want to know is how to cope and how to get better, not how to prevent something that has already happened. But you *do* need to read this chapter, for you are about to become one of the most effective advocates of burn prevention. No one knows better than you and your family the anguish that a major burn can cause, and for this reason it is natural for you to become an activist in burn prevention. Our hope is that you can stop someone else from experiencing what you have experienced.

This chapter describes the principles of prevention. Each and every one of us in our daily lives and in our homes is guilty of breaching one or more of the principles of burn prevention. The American Burn Association is the only professional association trying to run itself out of business, by teaching prevention and abolishing burns. You can help to do this by spreading the message in this chapter.

Inside the Home

Most burn injuries—85 percent of them—occur in the home, more often in the kitchen, bathroom, and bedroom than anywhere else. Scalds, electric burns, chemical burns, and injury from fire occur in homes across the country every day. But almost all of these injuries could be avoided if burn prevention measures were taken. In the following section, we identify hazards in specific areas of the house and tell you how to eliminate them.

To protect your family from burn injury in the home, we suggest that you go through your home and make a list of the hazards you find. Then assign duties for each member of the household, and determine a schedule for completion of the tasks necessary to correct the problem. A week or so later, take a second tour of the home and make certain that all of the hazards have been eliminated.

To protect your family from the serious injuries that result from a house fire, get everyone together for a fire safety check in and around your home. Practice exit drills from each room in your home. You should have *two* escape plans for each room, especially the bedrooms (see the description of EDITH—Exit Drills in the Home—in this chapter).

Make sure that overnight visitors to your home as well as babysitters and other caregivers know the safety rules and fire escape plan for your household. If you are leaving your home and children in the care of someone else, make certain those caretakers know how to reach you, how to reach the police and fire department (post the number by the telephone, even if the number is 911), how to reach a friendly neighbor, and how to reach the children's doctor. Babysitters should take a first aid course and should read Appendix A in this book. They should look in on the children frequently and should not play the television or radio so loud that they cannot hear the children.

Tell your babysitters what to do if a fire starts. They should first get everyone out of the house—and no one should reenter the house having once left it. If the babysitter or the children catch fire, they should stop, drop, and roll: stop where they are, drop or get down to the ground, and roll over and over until the fire is extinguished.

If they cannot rescue the children without endangering themselves, babysitters should go to the neighbor's house and call the fire department and then return to the outside of the house and tell the firefighters where the children are.

A few words need to be said about children and toys. Matches, lighters, cooking utensils, and so on belong to Mom and Dad, not to the children. Consider that the child who is pacified by being allowed to play with a lighter may take that lighter and run it along a carpet or towel, causing the material to ignite. Or that the child who has in the past been given a kitchen pot to bang on may one day reach up and grab a hot pot off the stove, thinking it is a toy. Children have their toys and you have your tools. Keep them separate.

Nor do children need "cigarette lighter squirt guns" or "gasoline can piggy banks." If you believe, as we do, that these "look-alike toys" give children a false sense of security about something that is actually very dangerous, you might consider writing to the manufacturers to voice your displeasure with their product, or asking the store manager to reconsider whether stocking these items is a good idea.

The kitchen

1. Children should be continually supervised while in the kitchen. Establish an "off-limits section" or a "'no' zone" around cooking areas, the oven, the microwave, and the toaster oven. This area can be marked off with masking tape on the floor, or a floor mat can be used.
2. Keep pot handles turned inward. Use potholders or oven mitts, especially when handling pots with metal handles.
3. Dish towels were not meant to be used near the stove. Keep curtains, aprons, dish towels, and other flammable items away from the stove.
4. Secure loose sleeves with an elastic band while cooking.
5. Always attend food while it is cooking. *Do not* leave the house.
6. Only use Underwriters' Laboratory (UL)–approved appliances. Do not allow cords to dangle off countertops. Unplug all small appliances when they are not in use.
7. Oil and grease catch fire quickly. When cooking with these substances, watch closely for smoke and spattering of oil or grease from the pan or deep fryer.
8. Keep the inside and outside of the stove as well as the hood clean of grease. Accumulated grease can ignite.
9. Do not throw water on a grease fire; water will spread the fire. When cooking in a pot, keep an appropriate lid at hand to cover the pot in case of a fire. Leave the lid on for at least 15 minutes. If the fire reignites, cover it again and call the fire department. Baking soda is a good extinguishing agent. Never use flour, cornstarch, baking powder, or sugar on a fire.
10. If a pot boils over and puts the gas burner out, turn the burner off and wait a few minutes before relighting.

11. The back of the stove should only be used to hold nonflammable decorative items. Cookies and treats for children and salt and pepper and other condiments should not be stored above or behind the stove.

12. Place toaster ovens and toasters on a hard surface; do not place a tablecloth or paper towels under any appliance that heats up. Do not store anything on top of a toaster oven.

13. If you suspect a gas leak, leave the area immediately and call the gas and electric company from a neighbor's house.

14. Before going to bed, make sure the burners and the oven are turned off.

Microwave Ovens. Microwave ovens are handy kitchen appliances, but they must be used properly. Among the greatest hazards in microwave use are bottleneck containers such as baby bottles and syrup bottles. As the liquids heat in these containers, steam is caught under the lip of the container. Since the microwave oven heats quickly, the steam has little time to escape, and the liquid in the bottle can violently erupt. This eruption can occur when the bottle is in the oven, immediately after it is taken from the oven, or as the bottle is tipped over, to feed the baby, for example.

Hot milk from an erupting bottle can cause a third-degree scald burn in an infant. A 4-ounce bottle of formula at room temperature (75°F), when heated in a microwave oven, reaches a temperature of 165°F in just 60 seconds. (Smaller amounts heat more rapidly.) *Never heat a baby's milk or formula in the microwave oven,* unless it is specifically packaged for the microwave.

Follow the precautions listed here to avoid burn injury from microwave use.

1. Install the unit properly: level the oven and allow space for ventilation. If you don't have a copy of the installation and use instructions, send the model number to the manufacturer and obtain them.

2. If the unit is dropped, have it checked. (If the door's seal is broken, microwaves can escape.) Periodically check the cord for damage.

3. Only an authorized person should repair the microwave.

4. Keep the oven clean with nonabrasive cleaners. Leftover food particles will refocus the microwaves and may cause damage.

5. Children who use the oven should be tall enough so that their face is not directly in front of the oven chamber when the door is open. Generally, children under the age of seven should not be permitted to use the microwave oven.

6. The microwave oven is not a dryer. Do not attempt to use it to dry clothes or other articles.

7. Use only microwave-safe containers in the microwave. Read and follow warnings on cooking containers. Some containers are used for cooking. Others are meant to be used only to reheat foods.

8. Metal-trimmed glassware or china cannot be used in the microwave oven. The gold or silver will refocus the microwaves. A cup or mug with metal trim can burn your lip.

9. Some manufacturers approve the use of small strips of aluminum foil to protect certain areas of the food from overcooking (such as the turkey wings and drumsticks). Some state that it is safe to defrost turkeys without removing the metal clamps first.

Defrosting is generally done at a lower setting. Metals reflect microwaves, and heating metals in a microwave can lead to arcing and sparks. Should this happen, stop the power.

10. Only use twist ties that are approved for microwave use. Twist ties that have a piece of metal in their center should not be used.

11. Use caution when heating liquids in containers with a smooth surface. The liquids heat faster, and the slightest movement or addition to such a container can cause an eruption.

12. Only use plastic wraps that are designed for microwave use.

13. It is dangerous to operate an empty microwave. To avoid doing so inadvertently, or having a child do so, keep a microwave-proof cup filled with water in the chamber or unplug the unit.

14. Scald burns are the most frequent burns associated with microwave cooking. Keep an oven mitt or potholder handy to use when removing foods or containers from the unit.

15. Steam must have an escape route. Place lids on loosely and leave an opening in the plastic to avoid an eruption. Slit pouches containing food (except popcorn) before putting them in the microwave. Pierce all solid vegetables (such as squash and potatoes) with a fork before cooking. They can rupture in the oven too, as the skin acts like a sealed pouch.

16. Steam from popcorn bags can burn the eyes and face. Turn the bag away from your face as you open it.

17. The moisture content in the various parts of a food creates different temperatures within the same heating time. For example, the jelly in a doughnut becomes very hot (more moisture and sugar), while the outside (less moisture) stays cooler.

18. Let the foods "rest" in the oven before removing them. This will allow the pressure from the steam to decrease.

19. Use a fork to lift the container's lid or remove plastic coverings. Keep the mitt on in case the container slips.

20. Do not lean over the hot container. Steam may escape and injure your eyes.

21. Make additions to the food with caution. Some additions, such as salt, instant coffee, and a cold spoon, can cause an eruption.

22. Stir foods to distribute heat. Microwaves cook food from the outside to the inside. The moisture closest to the outside is heated first. The inside cooks as the heat is conducted toward the center. Containers become hot when the food conducts heat to the container.

23. Pierce egg yolks with a fork or toothpick; remove the shell.

24. Starting temperatures make a difference in the total cooking time. Frozen foods take longer than those at room temperature. Make adjustments.

25. Make a depression in the center of thick foods such as mashed potatoes to allow for more even heat distribution and safer cooking.

26. Never leave a microwave oven unattended.

The bathroom

1. Hot-water heaters should be set no higher than 120°F to decrease the chance of scald burns.

2. Whenever you use water, turn on the cold water first and then gradually add hot water.

3. Baby's bath water temperature should not be over 100°F. Test the water temperature before placing the child in the tub. Don't put the child in the tub until the water has been turned off. Never leave a child unattended in the bathtub.

4. Keep hair dryers, curling irons, and other electrical appliances away from water and water sources. Unplug appliances after each use. After bathing, dry off before using these appliances.

The bedroom

1. Never smoke in bed.
2. Place beds, especially children's beds and cribs, away from heaters, electrical outlets, stoves, fireplaces, and radiators.
3. Dress children in fire-retardant sleepwear.
4. Don't use a heating pad or hot-water bottle when you are ready to go to sleep.
5. Install smoke detectors outside the bedrooms. (Being warned after the fire has reached the bedroom is too late.)
6. Close the bedroom door before going to sleep. This will help keep smoke and flame from entering the bedroom.
7. Do not fold or roll an electric blanket; don't lie on top of an electric blanket.
8. Only purchase UL-approved heating equipment.
9. Follow the manufacturer's directions for use of all heating equipment.

The living room

1. Use deep ashtrays when smoking, and put them on a table. Never put an ashtray on the arm of a chair.
2. Place furniture away from stoves and heaters. Arrange furniture with an escape route in mind. Don't block your escape route with furniture.
3. Purchase furniture that is fire resistant.

The dining room

1. If young children will be dining with you, or if you will be burning candles, do not use a tablecloth.
2. Always test the temperature of liquid or solid food before feeding an infant or child (or anyone else who cannot test the temperature for himself).
3. Keep food close to the center of the table, not at the edges.
4. Make sure candles are extinguished before leaving the table.

The basement, garage, attic, and other storage areas

1. Keep these areas free from clutter.
2. Never lock the door between the house and a basement, garage, or other storage area.
3. Put oily rags *outside*, in a covered trashcan, and put them out for trash pickup. Do not store them.
4. Never store newspaper in a warm, damp place. It can self-ignite.
5. Keep the basement door closed at night.
6. A basement door that is at the head of a stair must fit tightly in the jamb, to help contain a fire that starts in the basement.

Heating systems

Space heaters

1. Purchase only UL-approved space heaters.
2. Place space heaters at least 3 feet away from furniture, curtains, play areas, and exit paths.
3. Purchase only a freestanding space heater that has a tip-over switch. This switch will automatically shut the heater off if the heater is knocked over.
4. Make sure there is a guard around the coil of the heater.
5. Never use a space heater in the same room where gas or other volatile liquids are being used or stored.

Fireplaces

1. Make sure wood is dry. Don't use wet or damp wood. (See Table 8.1. for firewood ratings.)
2. Never use flammable liquids in the fireplace.
3. Do not burn household trash in the fireplace.
4. Dispose of *cool* ashes in a metal container.
5. Keep the damper open and the glass door of a fireplace closed when in use.
6. If the fireplace doesn't have a glass door, keep a screen over the opening.

Table 8.1. Ratings for Firewood

	Relative amount of heat	Easy to burn	Easy to split	Heavy smoke?	Pop or throw sparks?	General rating and remarks
Hardwood trees						
Ash, red oak, beech, birch, hickory, hard maple, pecan, dogwood	High	Yes	Yes	No	No	Excellent
Soft maple, cherry, walnut	Medium	Yes	Yes	No	No	Good
Elm, sycamore, gum	Medium	Medium	No	Medium	No	Fair—contains too much water when green
Aspen, basswood, cottonwood, yellow poplar	Low	Yes	Yes	Medium	No	Fair—but good for kindling
Softwood trees						
Southern yellow pine, Douglas fir	High	Yes	Yes	Yes	No	Good but smoky
Cypress, redwood	Medium	Medium	Yes	Medium	No	Fair
White cedar, western red cedar, eastern red cedar	Medium	Yes	Yes	Medium	Yes	Good—excellent for kindling
Eastern white pine, western white pine, ponderosa pine, true firs	Low	Medium	Yes	Medium	No	Fair—good for kindling
Tamarack, larch	Medium	Yes	Yes	Medium	Yes	Fair
Spruce	Low	Yes	Yes	Medium	Yes	Poor—but good for kindling

Source: U.S. Department of Agriculture, Forest Service, Leaflet No. 559 (1974).

7. Never throw charcoal or Styrofoam into a fireplace.

8. If a fire starts in a fireplace or wood-burning stove, do not close the damper.

9. The front hearth should extend at least 20 inches in front of the fireplace opening and must be made of fireproof material.

10. Do not place rugs or furniture within 3 feet of the front of the fireplace.

11. Rugs and floor coverings close to the fireplace should be made of fire-resistant material.

12. Have your chimney cleaned at least once a year.

13. Do not use fans in the house when there is a fire in the fireplace.

14. Be sure there is plenty of oxygen to feed the fire; if necessary, open a window slightly.

The furnace

1. At the beginning of each heating season have your furnace inspected for potential hazards such as clogged outlets or leaks.

2. Furnaces should be installed away from walls and ceilings.

3. Ducts and filters need to be cleaned several times a year. Make sure the unit is turned off before cleaning.

4. If the furnace doesn't start, call a professional.

5. Never use kerosene or other flammable liquids to start a fire in a coal furnace.

6. Make sure the ceiling above a basement furnace is covered with plaster or a plasterboard. If the ceiling or dry wall near a furnace feels hot, additional insulation is required.

7. If a fire starts in a furnace, radiator, or water heater, shut off the power immediately.

Electric supply in the home

Electric outlets and power cords

1. Ground-fault interrupter (GFI) circuit breakers or receptacles should be installed if the receptacle is within 7 feet of a sink or wet area. This is a requirement of the safety code in some states.

2. Insert outlet covers into unused outlets to keep children's fingers out of them.

3. Keep all electric cords out of reach of children and pets and away from heating elements and burners.

4. Extension cords should be used only as a temporary solution. If you must use an extension cord, use a "power strip" with a 15-amp circuit breaker. Keep extension cords in good working order. Remember, match the load of the cord to the job.

5. Do not run cords under rugs, through door jams, behind radiators, across sidewalks, or over nail heads, as this will damage the cord.

6. Always remove a plug from the outlet by grasping the plug and pulling straight out. Yanking on the cord will damage the connection inside the plug.

7. It is not necessary to use a three-prong power cord or a grounding system with double-insulated electrical equipment, which has two layers of insulation. This equipment should be repaired only by an authorized repair shop.

8. Do not remove the third prong on a three-prong plug. This is the ground wire, and it is necessary to prevent electrocution and overload when using electrical equipment that is not double insulated.

9. Frequently blown fuses are a warning. Check with your electrician or power company before using a different fuse.

10. If you are not trained in electrical safety, call an electrician. Some insurance companies will not honor your claim if an unqualified or unlicensed individual did the work.

Aluminum wiring. Call a qualified electrician to inspect the wiring in your home if you notice any of the following warning signs:

1. Face plates on outlets or switches are warm to the touch.
2. Lights flicker.
3. Outlets or switches smell like burned plastic.
4. Circuits don't work.

Safety Devices and Fire Escape Plans

Smoke detectors

1. We recommend that you install at least one smoke detector on every level of your home.

2. If your bedrooms are all located on the second floor of your

home and you are only installing one smoke detector, it should be installed close to the bedrooms but between the bedrooms and the rest of the house.

3. You should sleep with your bedroom door closed. For this reason, it is a good idea to install an extra smoke detector inside your bedroom.

4. It is a good idea to install a smoke detector in trouble-spot rooms, such as rooms where people regularly smoke.

5. Install smoke detectors at least 6 inches away from where the wall and the ceiling meet.

6. Do not install smoke detectors next to heating and cooling vents.

7. Check your smoke detectors' alarms every month according to the manufacturer's instructions.

8. Replace smoke detector batteries at least once a year. An even better idea is to replace them every spring and fall at the same time you reset your clocks for daylight savings time. It is a good idea to vacuum your detectors at this time to remove dust and cobwebs.

9. Use alkaline batteries in smoke detectors; they have a longer shelf life.

10. If the "low-battery" warning chirp goes off, do not just take the battery out of the smoke detector—replace it immediately. Keep extra batteries stored in the refrigerator for this purpose.

11. Never let anyone borrow the batteries from your smoke detector.

12. If you have been gone from your house or apartment for a short period of time, check your detectors when you get home to be sure you were not away at the same time your low-battery chirp went off.

13. If your smoke detector sounds the alarm because of cooking smoke, do not take the battery out. Fan the smoke away. These false alarms can be avoided by relocating the smoke detector or buying one with a delay switch.

14. Don't buy smoke detectors that run on household electric current only. They will not work during power failures. If you own this kind of detector, always provide a battery backup.

15. Take malfunctioning detectors to the store immediately.

16. Follow maintenance instructions that come with your detector, especially photoelectric detectors.

Fire extinguishers

1. Purchase only UL-approved fire extinguishers.

2. Make sure that you are strong enough to lift and operate an extinguisher before buying it.

3. There are different classes and types of fire extinguishers for different classes and types of fires. Install several multipurpose fire extinguishers in particularly hazardous areas of the home, such as near the stove (but by the room's exit), near the furnace in the basement, and in any area where flammables are stored.

4. Extinguishers must be recharged after every use. When you buy a fire extinguisher, ask your dealer how it should be inspected and serviced.

5. Read the directions and learn how to properly use your fire extinguisher at the time of your purchase.

6. Do not start to fight a fire with an extinguisher until you are sure everyone has exited the building and the fire department has been called.

7. Do not fight a fire with an extinguisher if you cannot operate the extinguisher without reading the directions first or if you are not sure whether the extinguisher is large enough or the right class or type to fight the fire.

8. Never try to fight a fire if it has started to spread or is already a large fire.

9. Abandon attempts to fight a fire if the fire could block your escape route.

10. Replace disposable fire extinguishers after they have been used.

11. A home sprinkler system, though costly, is usually an effective extinguishing device. Check your local building codes before proceeding.

Escape: EDITH

1. Draw a diagram of your house or apartment. Include every room, hallway, stairwell, door, and window. On your diagram, mark at least two exits out of every room.

2. Conduct periodic *E*xit *D*rills *I*n *T*he *H*ome (EDITH). These drills increase the chances of surviving a dwelling fire.

3. Teach children not to hide from fire where firefighters cannot find them.

4. Make sure all windows and doors can be opened quickly. If you have bars on your windows or deadbolt locks, make sure they can be unlocked from the inside, that the keys are close by, and that every household member knows where the keys are.

5. Escape ladders for second-story rooms are a good investment.

6. Make it a habit to keep hallways and exits clear of objects.

7. If you are alerted to a fire by smoke or a smoke detector, don't panic but don't stop to pick up anything, either.

8. If the fire is in your room, get out quickly, closing the door behind you.

9. If the fire is not in your room, first feel the door to see if it is hot. Start from the bottom and go up to the top. If the door is not hot, stay low behind the door with your body pressed against it. Slowly unlatch the door, being prepared to slam it shut again in the event of heavy smoke or fire. If you don't feel any pressure pushing the door, open it a small amount and check for smoke. Do this a little at a time until you are sure it is clear enough to check the hall or adjoining area. If it is clear, stay as low as necessary to avoid smoke, cover your face with a moist cloth if possible, and go quickly toward the exit.

10. Do not use an elevator during a fire.

11. Scream or shout as loud as possible to alert the rest of the household to the fire.

12. Once you have escaped the building, you can call the fire department from a public phone or a neighbor's house. Or you can pull the fire alarm box, if there is one on your street.

13. Meet the members of your household at a prearranged spot out of the pathway that emergency vehicles will use.

14. Do not go back into a building that is on fire for any reason. Report trapped people and pets to the fire department immediately.

15. If smoke or fire has trapped you in your room, close all doors to the room and seal off the cracks under them with moist towels, rags, rugs, etc.

16. Cracks around doors and vents can be sealed off with duct

tape that is at least 2 inches wide. Keep a roll of duct tape in every room.

17. Dampen a cloth to keep your mouth and nose covered to help you breathe easier. *It is a good idea to keep a container of water in every room.*

18. Carefully open the window far enough to hang a bright piece of cloth or sheet or to wave a bright object, such as a flashlight, to attract attention, and then close the window to avoid venting smoke or fire in the room from the outside.

19. If there is a phone in your room, call the fire department to let them know that you are trapped and where you are located in the building.

20. Stop, Drop, and Roll. If you should catch on fire, do *not* run. **Stop** where you are, **drop** or get down to the ground, and **roll** over and over until the fire is extinguished.

Reporting a fire

1. Just as you should practice your escape plan, you should practice properly reporting a fire.

2. Keep the telephone number of your fire department posted by all of your telephones where it can be easily found when needed.

3. Try to be as accurate as possible when reporting the address of the location of a fire. Reporting "20 Dogwood Street" when the address is "20 Dogwood Road" could cause an undue delay in response time. Speak clearly and don't hang up until the fire department does.

4. Try to give a brief description of the nature of the fire. For example, you might say, "I'm calling to report a fire in a multiple-family dwelling. Flames are shooting out of the third-story window."

5. Teach your children their street name and number at as early an age as possible.

Special Considerations in the Home

Smoking

1. Ashtrays should be large and deep, and they should not have notches on the side.

2. Don't smoke alone.

3. While smoking, keep a cup of water close by.

4. Install a smoke detector in rooms that are frequently used by smokers.

5. Keep ashtrays away from combustible materials.

6. Do not use flammable or combustible products such as hairspray while smoking.

7. Use a steady table, not your lap or the arm of your chair, to hold your ashtray.

8. If you drop a lit cigarette into a sofa or chair, find it and remove it immediately. Make sure the upholstery has not started to smolder or burn.

9. Make it a habit to check in and around chairs and sofas for cigarette butts before leaving a room where people have been smoking.

10. Wet cigarette butts with water before emptying an ashtray into the trash can.

11. Never smoke in bed or while reclining in a chair.

12. Be extra careful if you smoke when you are tired, while drinking alcoholic beverages, or when taking medicine that could make you drowsy.

13. Supervise elderly or impaired persons when they smoke, particularly persons whose motor ability is impaired (such as stroke victims) and persons who are bedridden.

14. Adhere to all smoking ordinances and policies.

15. Obtain permission from the staff of a nursing home or hospital before giving smoking materials to the person you are visiting.

Matches and lighters

1. Do not leave matches and lighters in easy access areas such as in purses, on tables, and in home decorations. Store them high, out of children's reach. Do not store them around flammable materials or in damp areas.

2. Do not keep wooden strike-anywhere matches in homes where there are young children.

3. Avoid using matches that have been exposed to dampness or look as if they have been damaged or discolored.

4. Empty pockets of matches and lighters before storing clothes for the season. Safely dispose of old matches.

5. Do not pack matches or lighters in luggage.

6. Close the cover before striking a match and strike it away from yourself and others. Stay away from faces or fabrics when striking a match. Never strike a match around any flammable liquids or vapors or any volatile chemicals of any kind.

7. After striking a match, hold it long enough to be sure it is out and dispose of it properly.

8. Before putting them back in your purse or pocket, make sure the lid is tightly closed on lighters that burn until the cover is closed.

9. Avoid spilling lighter fluid when filling the lighter. Never smoke while filling a lighter.

10. Teach young children, especially those three and younger, that matches and lighters are for adults only. You can positively reinforce this by rewarding them if they bring to you any matches or lighters they find.

11. When you feel your children are ready (suggested age is five years old), teach them that a match is a "tool" with a specific purpose. Teach them that matches should only be used for such purposes as lighting campfires and candles. Show them how to safely light a match. Let them light matches under your supervision until they do not desire to light any more.

12. Make an agreement with your child to allow them to light matches when it is appropriate, but only under adult supervision.

13. Do not give children lighters (even if they are empty) to play with. This teaches them that a lighter is a toy, not a tool. This includes car lighters.

14. Do not give a lighter to children as a substitute for matches to be used for such purposes such as camping and scouting activities.

Flammable liquids

Common flammable household liquids include gasoline, kerosene, lighter fluid, paint, paint thinner, and alcohol-based products. (See the section on gasoline use later in this chapter.) These liquids give off vapors that can catch on fire, sometimes from a spark or flame that is distant or out of sight. In order to avoid burn injury from the use of flammable liquids, follow these safety precautions:

1. Don't store or use flammable liquids near a pilot light or any source of heat. Fumes from these liquids build up and can ignite from a tiny spark.

2. Don't store any corrosive chemicals. Purchase enough for a one-time use and discard what you don't use.

3. Store all cleaning fluids in a metal container and away from any sources of heat.

4. An explosion can occur if vapors become concentrated in a confined area. Always use flammable liquids in a well-ventilated area.

5. The Federal Hazardous Substances Act established labeling categories for liquid consumer products that will burn. They are: *Extremely flammable*: produce ignitable vapors at room temperature or below. *Flammable*: produce ignitable vapors at greater than room temperature. *Combustible*: burn once they are ignited.

6. Some flammable products are not labeled as such because they are not flammable in liquid form as they come from the container. If products are not labeled, assume they are flammable.

7. Properly discard empty cans that once contained flammable liquids.

8. Never throw an aerosol can into an incinerator.

9. Use flammable liquids only for the purpose for which they were intended.

Flame-resistant and flame-retardant fabrics

1. Lightweight fabrics generally ignite more easily than heavier weaves.

2. By law, all children's sleepwear up to size 14 must be flame-resistant.

3. Use flame-resistant fabrics when making your own clothes, curtains, and so on.

4. Neither flame-resistant nor flame-retardant means that fabrics won't burn, so take extra care when wearing loose-flowing clothes to keep them away from flames or any sources of ignition (see Table 8.2).

Table 8.2. Fabric Flammability and Combustibility

Degree of Flammability				
Low 0		Medium 5		High 10
Asbestos Fiberglass	SEF Wool Nomex Kynol	Polyester Nylon FR cotton Other FR synthetics	Acetates Acrylics	Cotton Linen Polyester-cotton Rayon

Note: Many additional fabrics could be included here, but these indicate the degree of risk. Contact fabric manufacturers for information about a specific fabric.
FR = Flame Retardant
SEF = Self Extinguishing Fabric (trade name for a modacrylic made by Monsanto)

Outside the Home

Burn injury can occur as close to home as the backyard or the driveway. In the following section, we identify specific hazards outside the home and tell you how to deal with them.

An important consideration right outside your front door is the house number. The fire department needs to be able to find your house without delay, so your house number must be large enough to be clearly visible from the street. House numbers should be posted on a conspicuous background that is unobstructed. Three inches is a good size for letters and numerals for single-family residences. For multifamily homes and commercial and industrial buildings, letters and numerals 6 inches high are preferable.

Gardening and lawn care

These activities involve the use of chemicals and power tools (read the preceding sections on the use of electric power cords and flammable liquids). Observe these lawn-mowing safety rules:

1. Read and follow the safety sheet that comes with the device.
2. Wear safety glasses or goggles, solid-soled shoes, and long, snug-fitting pants. Open sandals, bare feet, and loose-fitting clothes are not appropriate. Extinguish all smoking materials while filling or operating a gas mower.

3. Do not remove or bypass the safety shields that are attached to weed trimmers and lawn mowers.

4. Clear the area of stones, sticks, wires, bones, and so on. If such an item is struck by a mower, it can become airborne and cause serious injury.

5. Allow damp or wet locations to dry before mowing or trimming.

6. Do not use electrical equipment in the rain.

7. Store equipment where it will remain dry and locked away from children.

8. Use only UL-approved outdoor extension cords. Select an extension cord of the appropriate length and gauge. Using an extension cord entails loss of power. Check your manual for recommendations.

Barbecuing

1. Follow the instructions packed with your grill.

2. Use outdoor charcoal grills or gas grills *only* outdoors. Toxic fumes can collect and cause death in enclosed areas.

3. Tie back long hair. Wear snug-fitting, natural-fiber clothes (synthetic materials melt or catch fire quickly).

4. Check the wind before lighting the fire. Position the grill so that cinders do not fly into your home or your neighbor's home, wash hung on clothes lines, dry grass, and so forth. If conditions are very windy, don't barbecue outside.

5. Place the grill away from the house (heat and cinders can catch under the eaves and start a fire or melt the siding). Place the grill off to one side, away from the traffic of people and pets. Keep children and pets away from the grill at all times. Keep the garden hose or a full bucket of water handy in case of an accident.

6. Use only approved lighter fluid for charcoal grills. Other flammable liquids can explode when lit. Research alternative briquette lighter methods at your neighborhood store. Never add charcoal lighter fluid to a fire once it has been lit. The flames can follow the fumes back up to the container.

7. Approach the grill from the side. Never open the lid with your face directly over the grill.

8. Use potholders and long-stem BBQ utensils when cooking. Potholders can burn and utensils can become extremely hot if left

close to the source of heat. Place them away from the source of heat.

9. Never leave the grill unattended while you are cooking.

10. Keep the grill clean. Leftover grease and debris can catch fire.

Protecting your home against arson

1. Install strong locks on all doors and windows in your home or business, but be sure that people can still escape from the building in an emergency. Don't use deadbolts that use a key on the inside.

2. Put up night lights around buildings.

3. Sheds or other buildings that contain flammable materials must be kept secure.

4. Be aware of the daily routine of your neighborhood so that you will notice if anything unusual occurs.

Lightning storms

Seek shelter indoors at the first sign of an approaching storm. If a lightning storm comes up suddenly, however, you need to take the following steps immediately.

1. Seek shelter indoors. If there is no other safe shelter, get into your car. The rubber tires are a ground for lightning.

2. If you are swimming or wading, get out of the water and seek shelter.

3. If you are boating, turn your boat to shore and get off the water. Always follow safe boating procedures: carry an emergency band radio and keep it tuned to a station that reviews offshore weather; wear your safety jacket; keep a waterproof flashlight and flares in the boat.

4. If you must remain outdoors, avoid flat, open areas and hilltops, and stay away from metal objects such as golf clubs, wire fences, and metal clothes lines.

5. Do not take refuge under a tree. Even if you are not hit directly, the current that passes through the tree can arc, making contact with you or setting your clothes on fire. Also, ground current can pass through the soil, creating a circuit between the ground and your legs which conducts electrical current.

6. If you are on the golf course, get in the golf cart. Again, the rubber tires offer some protection. Head for the clubhouse or shelter.

7. Once indoors, stay away from windows, open doors, and fireplaces. Unplug televisions, stereos, radios, hair dryers, and electric razors. Do not use electrical appliances such as washers, dryers, and stoves. Do not use the telephone or headphones. Do not take a shower or a bath.

Power transformers and power lines

1. Do not allow children to play on high-voltage transformers. Direct them to safer areas.

2. Teach children to look for wires running through trees and not to climb in these trees. Since electricity arcs, you can sustain a serious injury just by coming too close to power lines—you do not have to touch the lines to be injured.

3. If a model plane or kite is caught in the electric wires or a tree with wires running through it, call the power company to remove these items. The best alternative is to fly these items in an open field (never in a storm, of course).

4. Don't climb utility poles or towers, and don't allow you children to do so.

5. Report all downed wires to the power company immediately. Stay well away from these lines and anything hanging around them. Caution others to do the same.

6. Do not place swimming pools, wading pools, and decks beneath electric lines.

7. Call the utility company and cable company before digging (to plant trees and shrubs, lay underground lines, put in fence posts, etc.).

8. Do not plant trees where they may grow to interfere with power lines. The utility company has the right to cut trees back if they come close to power lines.

9. Leave room between the house and new shrubs or trees.

10. Check with the utility company in your area before planting around transformers and meters.

11. Some watering and fertilizing devices use probes. Do not use these devices around ground-level transformers or underground electrical service.

The automobile

1. Attend an automobile maintenance class for the novice. Some adult continuing education centers or community colleges offer such courses. Learn what you can do and what you had best leave to the experts.

2. Keep your car serviced and maintain a log.

3. Always wear protective gear (goggles, long pants, face mask) when working on your car, and keep a fire extinguisher rated for chemical and electrical fires, as well as a water hose, handy.

4. Allow the engine to cool before working on the radiator or exhaust system. Remove the radiator cap slowly, with a rag, while turning your face away from the engine. Turn the cap slowly. If the pressure is suddenly released, antifreeze and the superheated steam will violently escape and may cause a steam and a chemical burn.

5. Welding should only be done by trained and experienced persons. If the gas tank is not entirely empty and well ventilated, it can explode like a bomb when the welding torch is applied.

6. If you don't know how to prime a carburetor with gas, don't attempt it. Spilling gasoline on the engine can cause an engine fire.

7. If you do prime the carburetor with gasoline, put the gas can far away and stand back before the engine is started. Have your "helper" look for you to be in the clear before starting the engine. Keep the car door open so the person starting the engine can jump out in case of an accident.

8. Placing your hand over the air horn to choke the engine can result in a third degree burn. The backfire through the carburetor is extremely hot.

9. Gasoline has only one purpose: fuel for an engine (see below).

10. Before refilling a battery with acid, place a plastic bucket on the ground and under the battery area. Watch for drain-off: do not allow battery fluid to flow down the street. Keep a bucket of water or a water hose nearby. (Review the section in Appendix A on first aid for chemical burns before working with the battery.)

11. Although refrigerants used in air conditioners are not generally flammable, they can damage skin and the environment. Dealing with refrigerants requires specialized equipment for col-

lecting the gases should they escape. This is work for the expert.

12. Refrigerant gas plus the products of an open flame combine to make a poisonous gas called phosgene gas. Never weld in the same area where coolants are being used.

13. Refrigerants need room to expand when tanks are being filled or stored. Never completely fill the air conditioner tanks. As the heat increases, the tank can rupture and explode.

14. Before working on the electrical system, shut off the current. Use only insulated (full-length) screwdrivers when working on the automobile; they will protect you should you slip and hit an electric wire.

15. Connect jumper cables only in the proper sequence. Check your car manual before connecting. (Keep the manual in your automobile.)

Gasoline

The solvent properties of gasoline make it tempting to use gasoline as a cleaner for everything from paintbrushes to entire floors spattered with paint. *But gasoline is a fuel for engines; it should never be used as a household cleaner.* Table 8.3 provides a list of cleansers and their appropriate uses. Keep in mind that these alternative solvents are flammable, too, and that they must be used with caution. Open a container containing a flammable liquid only in a well-ventilated area. This reduces (but does not eliminate) the risk of explosion.

If the cleansers recommended in Table 8.3 don't do the job, we suggest that you call a local rent-all store, which can recommend equipment that will safely remove paint and other stubborn substances.

Explosions and burns caused by using gasoline to start or speed up a fire are familiar stories in any burn treatment facility. *Gasoline should never be used to start or fuel a fire.* There are many safe devices, such as starter blocks and electrical gadgets, for starting charcoal grills and fires in the fireplace. Investigate what's available at the neighborhood hardware store.

Using gasoline as an insect killer can cause a lawn fire. Sparks and arcs from electrical wiring can ignite the gasoline and burn the yard and house. *Gasoline should never be used as an insecticide.*

Table 8.3. Flammable Liquids and Their Uses

Flammable Liquid/Solvent	Flash Point* (°F)	Ignition Temp** (°F)	Uses
Gasoline	−45	536	Fuel for engines
Acetone	0	1000	Nail polish remover
Naphtha	28–85	450	Lantern/stove fuel Camping equipment
Methanol	52	867	Varnish remover/thinner
Turpentine	95	488	Paint remover/thinner
Stoddard solvent	100+	444	Cleaning agent solvent
Gunk (grease remover)	100+	494	Auto parts cleaner
Mineral spirits	104	473	Paint thinner/brush cleaner

*At this temperature, the substance gives off enough vapors to form an ignitable mixture with air (gasoline stored at −45°F produces sufficient vapor to burn, for example).

**Once ignited, the substance burns at this temperature.

The following principles help prevent burn injury when using gasoline.

1. Do not store gasoline near light switches, pilot lights, or a lawn mower. The vapors from gasoline can be ignited by a spark from any of these. Make sure that the gasoline storage area is ventilated.
2. Gasoline expands as it warms, so leave room in the container for expansion: fill three-fourths to four-fifths of the container. Don't overfill the car's gas tank, either, since the gasoline may spill as the tank heats up and the gasoline expands.
3. Store as small a quantity of gasoline as possible.
4. Do not store gasoline in the home or basement. Keep it in the shed or a secure storage box outside the home and away from direct sunlight.
5. Store gasoline in an approved container. Limit access to gasoline by children and arsonists by keeping the container out of reach and locked away. If this is not possible, purchase safety cans with a handle or spout lock.

6. Refuel engines (such as a lawn mower) only after the engine is cool.

7. Do not smoke while pumping or pouring gasoline.

8. Return the gas nozzle to its proper place after pumping gasoline. Check your gas cap and make sure that the gasoline hose is not wrapped around your bumper before you leave the area.

Away from Home

Burn injury has turned many a vacation or outing into a tragedy. Be aware of the following hazards when vacationing or boating.

Camping

Tents

1. Purchase only flame-resistant tents. "Flame-resistant" does not mean flameproof, so you'll still need to set up a safe distance from ignition sources—at least 15 feet from the cooking area, for example.

2. Never cook inside the tent or use gas lights or gas heating units.

3. Be on the lookout for wildfires. Keep a battery-powered radio with you and tune in for information. (Keep extra batteries on hand.)

4. Keep a knife handy inside the tent in case you need to cut your way out.

5. Always have a bucket of water handy for emergencies, no matter what type of cooking fire is used. Keep a fire extinguisher handy.

Campfires

1. Wear snug-fitting, natural-fiber clothes while building or tending a fire. Synthetic materials can melt. Secure long hair with rubber bands or pins.

2. Learn how to tell when it is safe to build a campfire. Call ahead for information on wind or drought conditions. There may also be pollution regulations. Call the forest rangers or park managers to find out whether you'll need permits.

3. Check the direction of the wind. Set up the cooking area so that the wind does not blow noxious fumes and cinders toward the tent or other living areas.

4. The popularity of campfires has depleted some areas of natural resources such as kindling and logs. Call ahead to find out about restrictions. Some areas will allow portable stoves even if campfires are not allowed.

5. Choose a cleared area away from foot trails, tree limbs, logs, leaves, stumps, tree roots. Clear to the bare ground.

6. If you need to clear sod from an area, save the sod: put it under a tree and water it occasionally. As you break camp, clear the cooking debris and replace the sod.

7. Clear the area for 3 feet around the edge of a campfire. This will ensure that the surrounding area will not catch fire.

8. Do not build fires on or under large stones. Large stones can be permanently scarred by the heat and soot of a fire.

9. Check beach regulations before starting a campfire on the beach. Some areas forbid the use of any open fire source. After a campfire on the beach, place used charcoal in designated containers. Never bury coals in the sand.

10. Visit your library for copies of Scouting and camping manuals. They offer valuable information about building campfires.

Camp stoves

1. Research different types of stoves. Choose one that is suitable for your needs.

2. Follow the manufacturer's directions.

3. Practice using the stove in your yard before going on your trip.

4. Make stoves "off limits" to children.

5. Use the appropriate fuel for your stove, and don't mix fuels.

6. Only refuel a cool stove, and only refuel a stove outdoors—never in the tent, the house, the garage, or any other enclosed area.

7. Overfilling the unit can cause flareup. Fuel spills can be avoided by using a funnel. Allow the funnel to dry in the air. Residual fuel can ignite.

8. If you spill the fuel on the ground, move the stove away from this area. The fuel on the ground can ignite and heat up the stove, causing an explosion.

9. Tighten the cap of the refill can and on the stove before lighting the burners.

10. Check all connections on hoses for a tight fit before lighting the burners.

11. Keep the stove clean. Leftover grease can ignite.

12. Check for clogged, cracked, or cut lines.

13. Some stoves have keys to regulate the flow. Immediately remove the key after use. The key will remain cool to the touch and can be used to readjust the stove during cooking.

14. Light a stove by approaching it from the side. Keep your head and hands off to the side by using long matches (like a fireplace match) or an extended lighter made for charcoal fires. Flareup can occur with these stoves.

15. If a pot is too heavy, it can damage a stove. A grill placed over the stove, with its own support, can decrease the danger presented here.

16. Do not leave the stove unattended.

17. Allow the stove to cool before packing up to leave.

18. Store fuel sources away from the cooking area and other heat sources.

19. Take the empty containers home with you for proper disposal or refilling.

20. Never throw a container—empty or not—into the fire.

21. If the containers are not a bright color, use brightly colored tape to identify them. You won't overlook them when you leave or mistake them for some other container.

Charcoal fires

1. Charcoal fires cannot be made on the ground: they need air to burn. If the camping area does not supply grills, use a portable grill. Grills can be made from a #10 can. Check the Scouting manuals in your local library for instructions.

2. Homemade or low-to-the-ground charcoal fire grills must be kept on cleared ground, just like campfires. Keep a bucket of water nearby.

3. Tinder and kindling are the safest natural charcoal starters. Check your neighborhood store for other devices (chimneys, blocks, candles).

4. Only use approved charcoal fluid. Other flammable liquids can explode and give off toxic fumes.

5. Never add charcoal lighter fluid to a fire once it has been lit. The flames can follow the fumes back up to the container.

Vacationing: motel or hotel

Fire prevention and precautions

1. Before you make your reservations, inquire about smoke detectors and sprinkler systems. Don't stay in a place that doesn't offer this kind of protection.

2. As soon as you arrive, familiarize yourself with the fire escape plans for your room. Locate this information on the room side of the door. There should be *two* plans of escape. Memorize both of them. Count the number of doors from your room to the exit. (It may be dark when you need to exit, and this information will help orient you.)

3. Know where the fire alarm is on your floor.

4. Keep your electric travel gear (electric razor, hair dryer) in safe working condition.

5. Report damaged wires, outlets, and appliances, as well as malfunctioning "EXIT" lights, to the management immediately.

6. Never smoke in bed.

7. Ask that food trays and carts be removed from your room. Do not place them in the hallway, where they could interfere with evacuation in the case of fire.

8. Keep coolers away from electric outlets.

9. Unplug all appliances before retiring for the night.

10. Before going to sleep, familiarize yourself with the room from the bed, so that you'll know in the dark which way to turn to reach the door. At your bedside before going to sleep, place a pair of soled, slip-on shoes and your coat or robe with your room key and a small flashlight in the pocket.

11. If you are away with family or friends, tell them how to prepare for a fire before retiring at night. Designate a meeting place outside the motel or hotel in the case of fire. (Don't choose a spot close to the entrance, where emergency equipment will parked.) Agree beforehand that if emergency personnel tell evacuees where to gather, group members are to leave their own spot and go to the professionally designated area instead.

In case of fire

1. In the case of a motel or hotel fire, do not stop to gather personal belongings.
2. If the fire is in your room, get out of the room, sound the alarm, and evacuate.
3. If you are in your room and the alarm sounds, put on your shoes and your robe or coat with the flashlight and key in the pocket. Go to the hallway door and feel it to determine whether it is warm.
4. *If the door is hot,* the fire may be on the other side of the door. *Do not open a door that is hot!* If the telephone works, call the fire department or outside operator. Let them know that you are trapped: state the hotel's name and your room number. Do not assume that the fire has already been reported by someone else. Place wet towels at the door to keep the smoke out. Wet your hair.
5. Shut off all appliances, including the air conditioning or heating. The ducts can carry smoke or invisible toxic fumes from the fire into your room.
6. Signal for help by placing a noticeable piece of fabric in the window. If you can open the window, hang the fabric out of the window and then close the window again. If the window is stationary, tie the cloth to whatever you can.
7. Do not leave the window open or break the window. The fresh air will fuel the fire and draw it to your location.
8. *If the door is cool* to touch, get low behind the unlocked door and press your body against it until the door feels unlatched. If there is no pressure (pushing the door against you), then open the door just a fraction of an inch and check for smoke. If you don't detect any smoke, open the door a little more and check again. If you still detect no smoke, slowly open the door wider, staying low to the ground, and check the hall or next room for clearance. If it is clear, cover your mouth with a cloth (wet if possible) and go low toward the outside exit. Close the door to your room behind you, to keep the air in your room from feeding the fire and to preserve the air in your room in case the way is blocked and you need to return to the room. This is also the reason for taking your key.
9. Remember which way you turn as you leave your room, and count the doors you pass.

10. Use the stairway. *Do not use the elevator in case of fire*: it could stop and its doors open onto the floor where the fire is, or it could jam, trapping those inside.

11. Go immediately outside and gather at your designated spot or where the emergency personnel direct you. Look for the members of your group. Report missing persons to the officials. *Do not go back into the building for any reason.*

12. If you have to turn back, remain calm. Try the second escape route. If it is blocked or the smoke is overpowering you, return to your room. Remember to count the doors; remember that these doors are on the other side of the hall on the way back.

13. Use your flashlight and/or feel for the room numbers. Once you reach your room, go inside and shut the door.

Boating

We recommend that you call the Department of Natural Resources in your state for a list of specific regulations and laws of boating. The following general rules apply:

1. Purchase a fire extinguisher that is appropriate for the size and construction materials of your boat.

2. Do not discharge any liquid or solid materials from your boat. Some of these materials are flammable and toxic, endangering other boaters and wildlife. You are required to report all spills to the Coast Guard.

3. When refueling a boat engine, make sure you close all doors, hatches, and ports to keep the gasoline vapors from settling in lower areas of the vessel.

4. Extinguish all sources of ignition before refueling.

5. After refueling, ventilate your boat before starting the engine.

6. Use only electric lights on the vessel. Do not use gas stoves, heaters, or lights on your boat.

7. Do periodic maintenance, or have your boat serviced, for clogged fuel lines, cracks, and rust areas.

8. Tell a reliable person that you are out on the boat, when you expect to return, and your port of departure. This person can alert the Coast Guard if you are overdue and in need of assistance.

During the Holidays

Fourth of July

1. All fireworks, whether legal or illegal, are dangerous.
2. We recommend attending a public fireworks display run by trained professionals rather then setting off fireworks at home.
3. When attending a public fireworks display, keep far enough away to avoid misfires or falling ashes, which can cause burn injuries.
4. Don't set off fireworks around dry grass.
5. Keep fireworks out of the reach of children.

Halloween

1. Purchase only costumes made of flame-resistant paper or fabric.
2. Loose and frilly costumes are more dangerous than snug-fitting costumes, since they are more likely to catch fire near an open flame.
3. Use flame-resistant materials to make decorations.
4. Never cover light bulbs with paper or cloth.
5. When lighting jack-o'-lanterns, use flashlights, not candles.
6. Keep cornstalk decorations away from fire.
7. Only visit haunted houses that have been inspected and licensed by local fire department officials.
8. Do not hold a private bonfire. Attend only bonfires that are controlled by local fire department officials.

Thanksgiving

1. Before beginning Thanksgiving Day cooking, make sure your stove and other equipment are in good condition.
2. After cooking, thoroughly clean grease from inside the oven and the stove.
3. Keep all flammable items (napkins, dried flowers, etc.) away from cooking appliances and table candles.

Christmas

The tree

1. Choose a tree that is fresh. Consider going to a tree farm and cutting it yourself to make certain that it is fresh. To check a cut tree for freshness, tap it on the ground: if many needles fall off, the tree is not fresh. You can also check the tree by bending the needles between your fingers: if they break, the tree is not fresh. Beware: some trees are sprayed green to make them look better.

2. If possible, keep the tree outside the house until you are ready to set it up.

3. Before placing the tree (in a tip-resistant stand), cut the trunk diagonally two inches above the first cut.

4. Pick a place away from all heat sources to set up your tree. Make sure it will not block traffic or exits. Water the tree daily.

5. Tie large trees off from at least two points to your wall or ceiling with strong wire.

6. External flameproofing treatments for trees are almost impossible to correctly apply at home and should not be relied on.

7. When many needles start to fall off the tree, it is time to dispose of the tree.

8. If you buy an artificial tree, make sure it is made of fire-resistant material.

Decorations

1. Use only UL-approved lights.

2. Do not hang lights from a metal tree, since this creates a source of serious shock injury. Use colored floodlights instead. Position the floodlights where children can't touch them, since they become very hot.

3. Each year, check all lights for bare or frayed wire, loose connections, and cracked or broken sockets. Discard or have repaired any that are not in perfect condition.

4. Never overload light circuits. Only string together the number of lamps specified in the instructions.

5. Never put more than three sets of lights on an extension cord.

6. Keep connection joints away from the tree's water supply.

7. Position lights on the tree so they do not touch needles or branches.

8. Install an on/off switch for lights away from the tree.

9. Keep light bulbs away from curtains and other flammable materials.

10. Do not use indoor lights outdoors. Use only weatherproof outdoor lights.

11. Remove outdoor lights as soon as the holiday season is over.

12. Unplug lights from the wall outlet before you go to sleep or leave your home.

13. To keep sparks from setting your tree on fire, do not run electric trains under it.

14. Use noncombustible or flame-resistant decorations and place them away from heat and electrical sources.

15. Use candles with caution, and never on or near the tree. Keep candles out of children's reach, out of windows, away from areas where they can be knocked or blown over, and away from flammable materials such as curtains.

16. Put candles in candlesticks before lighting them. Don't forget to blow them out before you go to sleep or leave your home.

17. Remove all decorations from around your fireplace before lighting a fire in the fireplace. Make sure the flue is open.

18. Do not burn wrapping paper or evergreen boughs in the fireplace; they burn rapidly and throw off sparks.

19. Follow the instructions included with your potpourri pot and exercise extreme caution when using it. Only use candles approved for use with a potpourri pot.

20. Never leave potpourri pots unattended when they are in use.

21. The candle flame is too close to your potpourri pot if soot forms on the bottom of the pot while it is in use.

22. As always, blow out the candles before going to sleep or leaving your home.

In the Workplace

Look around your workplace. You may have already identified potential hazards. Report and discuss these hazards with your supervisor or boss.

Invite a fire official trained in burn and fire prevention to come to your place of work to talk with employees and supervisors. The fire official can help plan fire drills and teach fire extinguisher safety and fire safety at the job site. Do you have a designated employee for each floor or area who has taken basic first aid or CPR training? What does the fire alarm sound like, and how should you exit your building in case of a fire? Have you been instructed on how to use a fire extinguisher—and do you know when you shouldn't use one? These are just a few questions to be discussed with the fire official. Make sure new employees receive this information.

Burn and fire prevention instructors keep current with new prevention developments by reading and attending classes. Let them share this information with you and your group in annual meetings with employees.

Safety tips for your specific workplace can be found in safety manuals, Job Safety Analyses (JSAs), company policies, and accident investigation reports from your local fire department or fire marshall. Other resources include your local OSHA office and the National Safety Council (444 N. Michigan Avenue, Chicago, Illinois 60611), ASSE (1800 East Oakton Street, Des Plaines, Illinois 60018–2187), and NFPA (Batterymarch Park, Quincy, Massachusetts 02269–910).

Health care facilities

1. Careless smoking is the most common cause of fire in health care facilities. Observe the smoking regulations at your institution, and never smoke where oxygen is present.
2. Practice routine fire drills.
3. Know where fire alarms, fire extinguishers, and fire hoses are located.
4. Participation in a fire safety class or in-service is mandatory.
5. Never use equipment that is unsafe. Check the condition of cords and equipment before beginning.
6. Keep combustible material away from heat-producing sources.
7. Store gas cylinders properly.
8. Keep the halls and stairs free from clutter.
9. Never wedge emergency exit doors open or closed.

10. Be sure the lighted "EXIT" signs are working properly.

11. Know how to shut off oxygen.

12. If a fire alarm sounds or you smell smoke, move all patients who are in immediate danger from flames or smoke. Close patients' doors and hall doors.

13. *In case of fire,* remember SAVE: *S*ave the patient; sound the *A*larm; *V*entilate; *E*xtinguish if possible (but only after the fire has been reported).

In the Neighborhood

Look for burn prevention education classes held throughout the year. For six consecutive years, the president has signed Senate Resolution 217, which declares the first full week of February as "National Burn Awareness Week." Burn professionals have used this week as the "kickoff" period for burn prevention, education, and awareness. (The National Burn Awareness Task Force together with 1991 California Senator Pete Wilson and 1991 Congressman Howard L. Berman [D-24th CA] have worked on these initiatives. Many thanks to them for their devotion and selflessness.)

Fire Prevention Week is in October of every year. Request information about either of these programs from your local fire department and school. Or contact your local fire marshall, government official, insurance company, or community leader. You can help us reach people through educational programs.

Appendix A

First Aid for Burn Emergencies

This appendix tells you how to act when there is a burn emergency. It presents a plan for providing first aid for the burn victim during the first few crucial minutes of injury. It tells you how to cope and what to do, as well as what *not* to do, until medical assistance arrives. The guidelines presented here emphasize safety for both victim *and* rescuer, because in order to be of assistance, the rescuer cannot become part of the emergency. Before you provide assistance to a burn victim, make certain it is safe to do so.

The information in this appendix is by no means a replacement for a complete first aid course or cardiopulmonary resuscitation (CPR) course. We urge you to register immediately to take such a course with the local office of the American Red Cross or the American Heart Association. Nor do the steps described here replace professional medical care. Anyone who has a second-degree burn or worse needs to be examined by a physician.

You may be the first person to respond to someone in need of help. Be sure that you can provide safe and competent first aid. Be sure that you will not create additional injury for the victim or for yourself. If you are the victim of an injury, you may be able to use your knowledge of first aid to direct someone else to care for you.

First-Degree Burns

1. Eliminate or remove the source of the burn (come in out of the sun, drop the hot object, etc.).
2. Gently remove any clothing that is over the burn.
3. Soak the burned area in cool water or take a shower, or apply cool compresses until discomfort is resolved.
4. DO NOT USE ICE on the burn.
5. Cover with a cool, moist, clean dressing.
6. Obtain medical advice if problems arise or if an existing serious medical condition exists.

Table A.1 What to Do in an Emergency

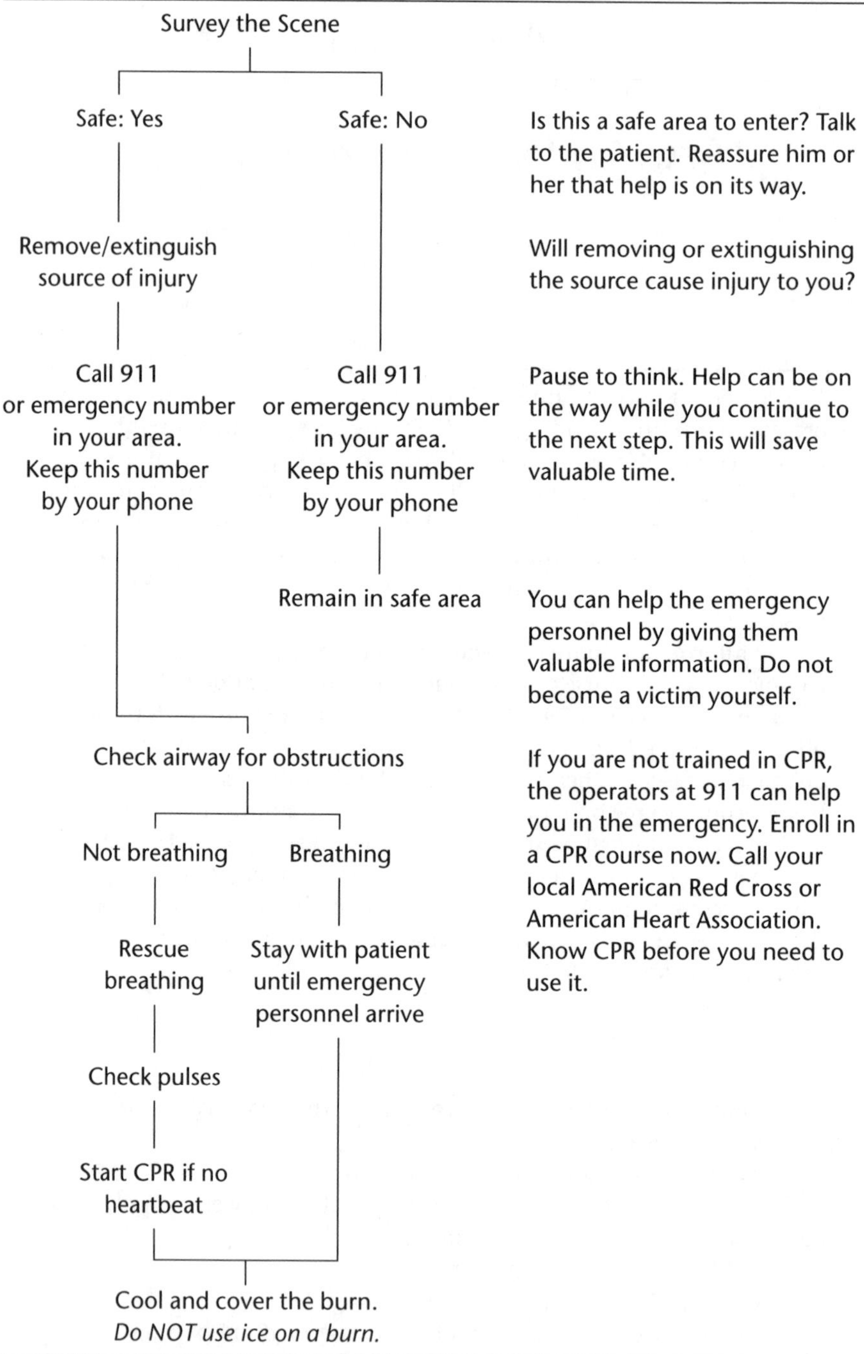

Second- and Third-Degree Burns

1. Survey the scene: is it safe for you to assist? If it is not—because of downed power lines or toxic chemical spills or another hazard—call for help immediately. Reassure the injured person that help is on its way.
2. If it *is* safe for you to help, your first step is to eliminate or remove the source of the burn.
3. Check to see if the injured person is breathing and has a pulse. If not, begin CPR if you have been trained in this skill. If the person is breathing and has a pulse, treat the burn.
4. Gently remove any clothing that is over the burn. If clothing is stuck in the wound, *do not pull it away*.
5. Cover with a cool, moist, clean dressing.
6. Do not use ice or over-the-counter ointments or creams.
7. Continue to reassure the victim.
8. Obtain medical care.

Remember: remain calm, and reassure the victim.

Chemical Burns

Survey the scene to determine whether you can reach the injured person without placing yourself in danger. Do not attempt to reach someone if you will be splashed with the chemical or overcome by fumes. You must wait for the arrival of professional personnel who are trained in chemical rescue.

Flushing a chemical requires plenty of water—gallons and gallons of water. Do not try to neutralize the chemical. Mixing acids and alkalines create heat, and this heat will cause even more skin damage.

Spilled dry lime presents a special situation. When water or any other liquid comes in contact with dry lime, the lime becomes active and starts to burn with a vengeance. To remove dry lime, gently brush it off the person's skin and clothing as well as out of the person's hair and scalp.

Remember, when dry powdery substances are brushed from any surface, the powder scatters in the air. Stand with any wind blowing the chemical away from you and the patient. Look to see that no one else is standing in the way. Ask the person to close his or her eyes before you brush off the dry lime.

Chemicals can splash into the eyes or seep through to the eyes. It is imperative that the eyes be flushed with a gentle, steady flow of water. If only one eye is involved, have the person tilt his or her head to the same side as the affected eye. This way the water will not run over into the uninjured eye. The flow should be from the nose to the ear. Don't forget to flush the face if it is also involved.

Table A.2 Chemical Burns

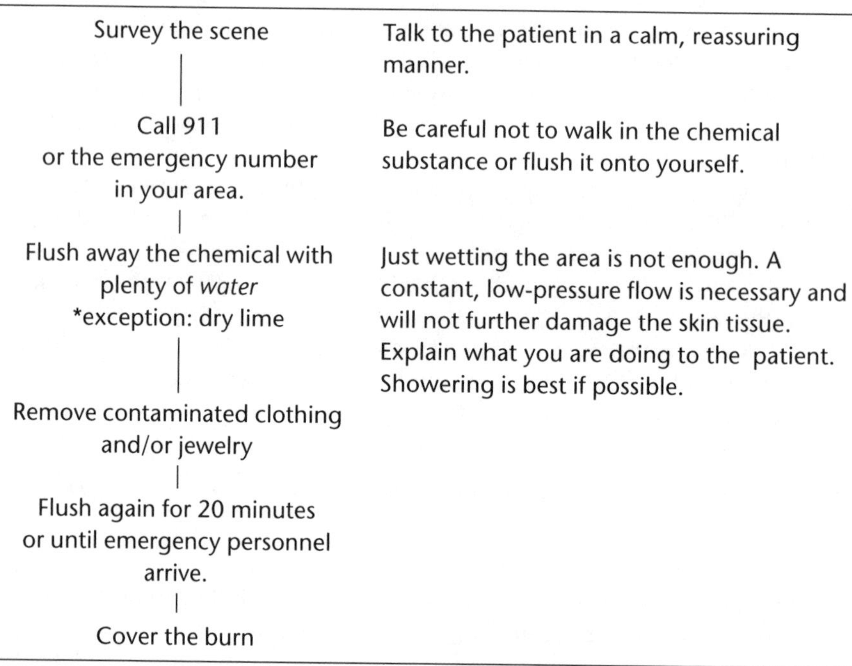

Step	Notes
Survey the scene	Talk to the patient in a calm, reassuring manner.
Call 911 or the emergency number in your area.	Be careful not to walk in the chemical substance or flush it onto yourself.
Flush away the chemical with plenty of *water* *exception: dry lime	Just wetting the area is not enough. A constant, low-pressure flow is necessary and will not further damage the skin tissue. Explain what you are doing to the patient. Showering is best if possible.
Remove contaminated clothing and/or jewelry	
Flush again for 20 minutes or until emergency personnel arrive.	
Cover the burn	

Flush for 20 minutes or more. If the patient complains of a burning sensation, flush again for another 5 minutes. Repeat this until the sensation of burning stops, or until emergency personnel arrive.

Smoke Inhalation Injury

When synthetic materials burn, they release fumes. These fumes may be visible as smoke, or they may be invisible. Both visible and invisible fumes from burning synthetic materials are toxic. Fumes, or gases, can overcome the healthiest of people. A piece of cloth placed over the mouth and nose may not adequately filter these gases. In the case of smoke inhalation injury, wait for the medical professionals to arrive if the situation is too dangerous to effect an efficient, quick, and safe rescue.

Because toxic fumes may interfere with the oxygen supply to the brain, a person may react violently to breathing in toxic fumes. This person will be strong and, very likely, combative. The person is not aware of what he or she is doing. Your role is to try to keep the person quiet and still. Remember: do not become part of the emergency. If help is not there and

Table A.3 Smoke Inhalation Injury

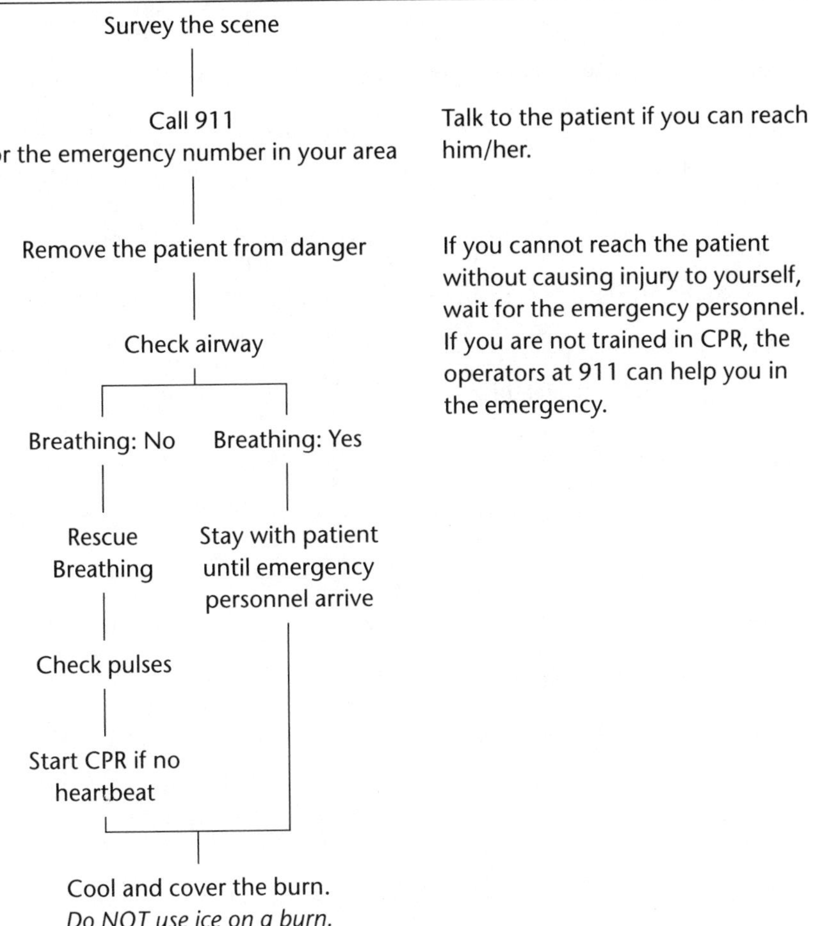

you cannot keep the patient in a sitting position without severely injuring yourself, you may need to limit your activities to watching the person, monitoring his or her actions until help arrives.

You must attempt to prevent the person from reentering the burning area.

Electrical Burns

Electrical burns can occur in the home or office as well as outside the home. If the emergency is outside and it is possible that downed power

Table A.4 Electrical Burns

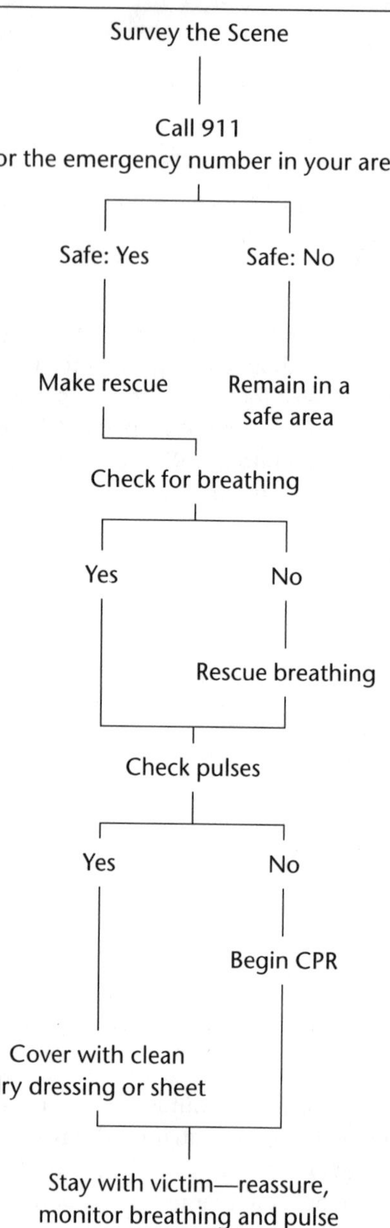

If you cannot safely effect a rescue without risking yourself, do not attempt a rescue. Wait for professional help to arrive. *Do not touch downed power lines.*

lines are in the area, *do not attempt to touch the victim*. Wait for professional help to arrive. If the accident occurs inside the home, turn off the power at the fuse box or circuit breaker. A dry, nonconductive material (such as a broom) can be used to break the victim's connection to the power source if the circuit breaker location is not known.

Electrical burns are usually deep injuries, involving second- and third-degree burns. With electrical burns, the possibility of cardiac arrest is also very real. As soon as you can do so safely, check to see whether the person is breathing and has a pulse. If not, begin CPR immediately if you have been trained in this technique. If the victim is breathing and has a pulse, treat the burn.

1. Turn off the power.
2. Survey the scene: is it safe for you to assist? If it is not, call for help immediately. Reassure the injured person that help is on its way.
3. Check to see if the injured person is breathing and has a pulse. If not, begin CPR if you have been trained in this skill. If the person is breathing and has a pulse, treat the burn.
4. Gently remove any clothing over the burn. If clothing is stuck in the wound, *do not pull it away*.
5. Cover wound with a cool, moist, clean dressing.
6. Continue to monitor pulse and breathing.
7. Continue to reassure the victim.
8. Obtain medical care.

Remember: remain calm, and reassure the victim.

Appendix B

Corrective Cosmetics for the Burn Patient

Corrective cosmetics can have psychotherapeutic value: cosmetics help many patients with the mental aspects of dealing with their disfigurement. Learning early on in the recovery stage about the uses and value of corrective cosmetics can promote the burn survivor's psychological well-being. Corrective cosmetics can also enhance the quality of life for patients; without this type of intervention, some patients voluntarily become social recluses and may be living what is considered a "societal death." But those who hide from life are missing so much. Life is about enjoying everything, from the simplest pleasures to the most luxurious. Empowering others to hinder your enjoyment in life is like letting them steal from you. You have already experienced a loss beyond your control, but remember: now you can try to control this new life and make the best of what you have. Corrective cosmetics allow many people to control their lives in a way they otherwise would not be able to.

The goal of the corrective cosmetic process is to re-create normalcy as closely as possible for individuals with skin discolorations or asymmetry problems. Skin discolorations (abnormal pigmentation) can result from all degrees of burn injuries. Asymmetry problems result from contractures (tightness of skin) or scars that change the contour of the skin surface. These problems can be camouflaged, or made less noticeable, with corrective cosmetics. Specialized techniques and materials can minimize the problems and help the burn survivor attain a normal appearance. This enhances the burn survivor's self-image, self-esteem, and social acceptance. The therapy is suitable for men, women, and children.

Corrective cosmetics used for burn survivors have special properties: high pigment concentration, tacky consistency, and staying power. The high concentration of pigment allows the makeup to provide coverage for any problem area. The tacky consistency helps the makeup adhere to burn-scarred or grafted skin, which is sometimes very smooth and slippery and which may have few (if any) pores into which the makeup can be blended. To achieve a very tacky texture and a high pigment concentra-

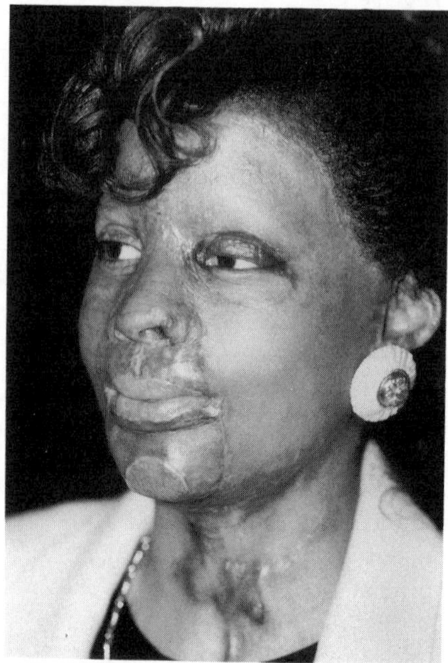
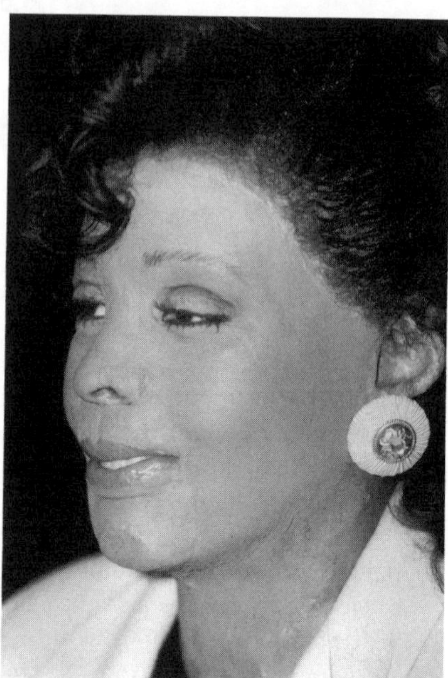

Figure B.1. Lawanda Conaway before corrective cosmetics and after.

tion, the makeup is usually creamy. The staying power of makeup for the burn patient is very important, however, so this creamy corrective makeup is set with a powder to create a more normal skin appearance and longer lasting wear.

Corrective cosmetics for the face are unique because they are focused on the most powerful source of non-verbal communication we have: the face is the primary medium through which we interact with the world around us. Corrective cosmetics facilitate that interaction for the burn survivor. Cosmetics empower the patient by reducing the patient's embarrassment as well as staring, strain, and pity from others. A patient is then able to shift attention to the person behind the face and define his or her own position instead of letting others define him or her with *their* behavior.

The face is not the only place where corrective cosmetics are applied. Almost all of the visual body parts can be treated with cosmetic therapy. Corrective cosmetics applied to the body allow the person to make clothing choices that may not have been possible without cosmetics.

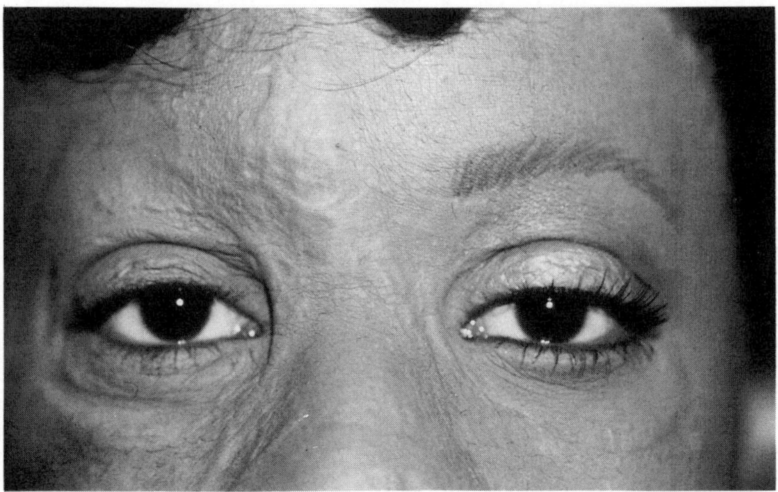

Figure B.2. Cosmetic reproduction of normal structure can minimize disfigurement. False eyelashes and penciled brow enhance the appearance of the area around the left eye.

In a corrective cosmetic consultation, the ease of application is always addressed. Whether the cosmetics will be applied by a novice at cosmetic application or a person with some skill at applying cosmetics or a person with limited physical functioning, the goal is to make the corrective cosmetic application an easy addition to everyday life. It is important for patients to remember that anything new takes practice to make perfect, and that applying makeup becomes easier with time.

The main concern of a program for corrective cosmetics is for the *patient's well-being*. In keeping with this philosophy, many product lines are used for patients, and generally no specific brands are endorsed. The only criteria used in selecting products is the products' ability to give effective results.

For more information about corrective cosmetics for the burn patient, contact Lawanda Conaway at the Center for Burn Reconstruction, the Francis Scott Key Medical Center, 4940 Eastern Avenue, Baltimore, Maryland 21224 (410-550-1090).

Appendix C

Burn Care Services in the United States and Canada

		UNITED STATES
Alabama	Birmingham	Children's Hospital of Alabama Burn Center 1600 7th Avenue, South Birmingham, AL 35233 205-939-9398
		UAB Burn Center University of Alabama Hospital 619 South 19th Street Birmingham, AL 35233 205-934-7250 205-975-5043 fax
	Mobile	University of South Alabama Burn Center 2451 Fillingim Street Mobile, AL 36617 205-471-7520 205-476-2806 fax
Alaska	Anchorage	Providence Hospital Thermal Intensive Care 3200 Providence Drive Pouch 6604 Anchorage, AK 99519-6604 907-261-3651 907-261-4884 fax

(*continued*)

Note: Adapted from *Burn Care Resources in North America, 1991–1992,* and *1993–1994* (American Burn Association). Used by permission.

Alaska (*cont'd*)

	Fairbanks	Fairbanks Memorial Hospital 1650 Cowles Street Fairbanks, AK 99701 907-452-8181
Arizona	Phoenix	Maricopa Medical Center Burn Unit 2601 East Roosevelt Street Phoenix, AZ 85008 602-267-5726 602-267-5450 fax
	Tucson	Carondelet St. Mary's Hospital Burn Unit 1601 W. St. Mary's Road Tucson, AZ 85745 602-622-5833 x4700 602-740-6069 fax
Arkansas	Little Rock	Arkansas Children's Hospital 800 Marshall Street Little Rock, AR 72202-3591 501-320-1323 800-367-2876 501-370-1139 fax
California	Berkeley	Alta-Bates Medical Center Burn Center 2450 Ashby Avenue Berkeley, CA 94705 510-204-1573 510-204-4380 fax
	Downey	Rancho Los Amigos Medical Center 7601 East Imperial Highway Downey, CA 90242 310-940-7454 310-940-6629 fax
	Fresno	Valley Medical Center Regional Burn Center 445 South Cedar Avenue Fresno, CA 93702 209-453-4561 209-453-5084 fax

Los Angeles	Children's Hospital of Los Angeles 4650 Sunset Boulevard Los Angeles, CA 90027-0700 213-669-2154 (days) 213-669-2120 (24 hours) 213-669-4106 fax
	Los Angeles County–University of Southern California Burn Center Ward 12-600, LAC–USC Medical Center 1200 North State Street Los Angeles, CA 90033 213-226-7991 213-226-5996 fax
Oakland	Children's Hospital of Oakland Burn Program 747 52nd Street Oakland, CA 94609 510-ICU-BURN (428-2876) 510-540-4380 fax
Orange	UCI Medical Center Burn Center 101 The City Drive Orange, CA 92668 714-456-5304 714-634-5690 fax
Sacramento	University of California Davis Medical Center Regional Burn Center 2315 Stockton Boulevard, T-5 Sacramento, CA 95817 916-734-3636 916-734-7411 fax
San Bernardino	San Bernardino County Medical Center 780 East Gilbert Street San Bernardino, CA 92404 714-387-8028

(*continued*)

California (*cont'd*)

	San Diego	Regional Burn Center University of California San Diego Medical Center 200 West Arbor Drive San Diego, CA 92103-6503 619-543-6503 619-293-0923 fax
	San Francisco	Saint Francis Memorial Hospital Bothin Burn Center 900 Hyde Street San Francisco, CA 94109 415-353-6255 415-353-6258 fax
		San Francisco General Hospital Burn Service–3A 1001 Potrero Avenue San Francisco, CA 94110 415-206-8201 415-206-5484 fax
	San Jose	Santa Clara Valley Medical Center Regional Burn Center 751 South Bascom Avenue San Jose, CA 95128 408-299-5242 408-295-8759 fax
	San Pablo	Brookside Burn Center 2000 Vale Road San Pablo, CA 94806 510-235-7006 x2789 510-215-5354 fax
	Sherman Oaks	The Burn Center at Sherman Oaks Community Hospital 4929 Van Nuys Boulevard Sherman Oaks, CA 91403 818-907-4580 818-907-4588 fax

	Stockton	Dameron Hospital Burn Unit 525 West Acacia Street Stockton, CA 95203 209-944-5550 x3542 209-466-3461 fax
	Torrance	Torrance Memorial Medical Center 3330 Lomita Boulevard Torrance, CA 90505 310-517-4622 310-784-4803 fax
Colorado	Colorado Springs	Penrose Hospital Burn Center 2215 N. Cascade Avenue Colorado Springs, CO 80907 719-630-5770
	Denver	The Children's Hospital Burn Center 1056 East 19th Avenue Denver, CO 80218 303-861-6516 303-861-3992 fax
		University Hospital University of Colorado 4200 East Ninth Avenue Denver, CO 80262 303-270-8052 303-270-8845 fax
	Grand Junction	St. Mary's Hospital and Medical Center 2635 N. 7th Street Grand Junction, CO 81501 303-244-2273 303-244-7510 fax
	Greeley	Burn Unit North Colorado Medical Center 16th Street and 17th Avenue Greeley, CO 80631 303-350-6570 303-350-6107 fax

Connecticut	Bridgeport	Bridgeport Hospital Burn Center 267 Grant Street Bridgeport, CT 06610 203-384-3728 203-384-3850 fax
	New Haven	Yale Burn Center Yale University School of Medicine (YPB 4) 333 Cedar Street New Haven, CT 06510 203-785-2876 203-785-5714 fax
District of Columbia	Washington	The Burn Center at the Washington Hospital Center 110 Irving Street, NW Washington, DC 20010 202-877-7241 202-877-3299 fax
		Children's Hospital National Medical Center Burn Unit 111 Michigan Avenue, NW Washington, DC 20010 202-745-5116
Florida	Gainesville	Shands Hospital Burn Intensive Care Unit 1600 S.W. Archer Road Gainesville, FL 32610 904-395-0200 904-338-9809 fax
	Miami	University of Miami–Jackson Memorial Medical Center 1161 NW 12th Avenue Miami, FL 33136 305-585-7085

	Orlando	Orlando Regional Medical Center 1414 South Orange Orlando, FL 32806-2093 407-841-5176 407-841-5111 x6421
	Tampa	Tampa Bay Regional Burn Center Tampa General Hospital Davis Islands P.O. Box 1289 Tampa, FL 33601 813-251-7141 813-251-7008 fax
Georgia	Atlanta	Grady Burn Center 80 Butler Street, SE Atlanta, GA 30335 404-616-3714 404-659-8620 fax
	Augusta	Humana Burn Center 3651 Wheeler Road Augusta, GA 30910 404-863-3232 800-241-5191 (GA) 800-241-5265 (Southeast) 706-650-6799 fax
		Medical College of Georgia Burn Unit 1120 15th Street Augusta, GA 30912 404-721-4721
Hawaii	Honolulu	Straub Burn Care Unit Straub Hospital 888 South King Street Honolulu, HI 96813 808-522-3731 808-522-4061 fax

Illinois	Chicago	Burn Center University of Chicago 5841 South Maryland Chicago, IL 60637 312-702-6736 312-702-5909 fax
		Sumner L. Koch Burn Center Cook County Hospital 1835 W. Harrison Street Chicago, IL 60612 312-633-6564
	Maywood	Foster G. McGaw Hospital/Loyola University Medical Center Burn Center 2160 South First Avenue Maywood, IL 60153 708-216-3988 708-216-8758 fax
	Rock Island	Trinity Medical Center Burn and Reconstructive Center 2701 17th Street Rock Island, IL 61201 309-793-3173
	Rockford	St. Anthony Medical Center 5666 East State Street Rockford, IL 61108 815-395-5313 815-395-5551 fax
	Springfield	Regional Burn Center Memorial Medical Center 800 North Rutledge Street Springfield, IL 62781 217-788-3325
Indiana	Fort Wayne	St. Joseph's Medical Center 700 Broadway Fort Wayne, IN 46802 219-424-BURN (2876) 219-425-3431 219-425-3432 fax

	Indianapolis	Indiana University Medical Center Burn Center Adult Burn Unit–Wishard Memorial Hospital 1001 West Tenth Street Indianapolis, IN 46202 317-630-6471 317-630-8721 fax
		James Whitcomb Riley Hospital Burn Unit (children) 702 Barnhill Drive Indianapolis, IN 46202-5124 317-274-3927 317-274-3404 fax
Iowa	Des Moines	Burn Intensive Care Unit Iowa Methodist Medical Center 1200 Pleasant Street Des Moines, IA 50309 515-241-5042 515-241-5351 fax
	Iowa City	University of Iowa Burn Treatment Center 200 Hawkins Drive Iowa City, IA 52242-1009 319-356-2496 319-356-8378 fax
	Sioux City	St. Luke's Regional Medical Center Burn Trauma Unit 2720 Stone Park Boulevard Sioux City, IA 51104 712-279-3440 712-279-3898 fax
Kansas	Kansas City	Gene and Barbara Burnett Burn Center University of Kansas Medical Center 39th and Rainbow Boulevard Kansas City, KS 66103 913-588-6142 913-588-7630 fax

(*continued*)

Kansas (*cont'd*)

	Wichita	St. Francis Regional Burn Center St. Francis Regional Medical Center 929 North St. Francis Avenue Wichita, KS 67214-3882 316-268-5388 316-291-7898 fax
Kentucky	Lexington	University of Kentucky Burn Unit Chandler Medical Center 800 Rose Street Lexington, KY 40536 606-233-5260 606-258-1949 fax
	Louisville	Humana Hospital–University of Louisville 530 South Jackson Street Louisville, KY 40202 502-562-3982 502-562-3446 fax
		Kosair-Children's Hospital P.O. Box 35070 Louisville, KY 40232-5070 502-629-5820 502-629-5769 fax
Louisiana	Baton Rouge	Baton Rouge General Medical Center Burn Unit 3600 Florida Boulevard Baton Rouge, LA 70806 504-387-7716 504-387-7088 fax
	Shreveport	LSU–Shreveport Burn Center LSU–Medical Center 1541 Kings Highway Shreveport, LA 71130 318-674-6850 318-674-6141 fax

Maine	Portland	Maine Medical Center 22 Bramhall Street Portland, ME 04102 207-871-2176 207-761-4294 fax
Maryland	Baltimore	Baltimore Regional Burn Center Francis Scott Key Medical Center 4940 Eastern Avenue Baltimore, MD 21224 410-550-0890 410-550-1165 fax
Massachusetts	Boston	Boston City Hospital 818 Harrison Avenue Boston, MA 02118 617-534-7395 fax Brigham and Women's Hospital Burn Center 75 Francis Street Boston, MA 02115 617-732-7715 617-566-9549 fax Shriners Burns Institute 51 Blossom Street Boston, MA 02114 617-722-3000 617-523-1684 fax Sumner Redstone Burn Center Massachusetts General Hospital Fruit Street Boston, MA 02114 617-726-3354 617-726-4127 fax
	Springfield	Baystate Medical Center 759 Chestnut Springfield, MA 01199 413-784-4800 413-784-5940 fax

(*continued*)

Massachusetts (*cont'd*)

	Worcester	University of Massachusetts Medical Center 55 Lake Avenue, North Worcester, MA 01655 508-856-5129 508-856-5250 fax
Michigan	Ann Arbor	University of Michigan Medical Center 1500 East Medical Center Drive Ann Arbor, MI 48109-0033 313-936-9666 313-763-0190 fax
	Detroit	Children's Hospital of Michigan 3901 Beaubien Boulevard Detroit, MI 48201 313-745-BURN (2876) 313-831-3908 fax
		Detroit Receiving Hospital Burn Center 4201 St. Antoine Detroit, MI 48201 313-745-3078 313-577-5310
	Flint	Franklin V. Wade Regional Burn Unit Hurley Medical Center #1 Hurley Plaza Flint, MI 48502 313-257-9188 313-257-9969 fax
	Grand Rapids	West Michigan Burn Unit 1840 Wealthy Street, SE Grand Rapids, MI 49506 616-774-7670 800-554-BURN (2876) 616-242-5193 fax
	Kalamazoo	Bronson Methodist Hospital Burn Center 252 Lovell Street Kalamazoo, MI 49007 616-341-6485 616-341-7574 fax

	Lansing	Regional Burn Center E. W. Sparrow Hospital 1215 East Michigan Avenue P.O. Box 30480 Lansing, MI 48909-7980 517-483-2647 517-483-2273 fax
	Saginaw	St. Mary's Medical Center-Burn Unit 830 South Jefferson Avenue Saginaw, MI 48601 517-776-8620
Minnesota	Duluth	Miller-Dwan Medical Center Burn Center 502 East Second Street Duluth, MN 55805 218-720-1215
	Minneapolis	Hennepin County Medical Center Burn Center 701 Park Avenue Minneapolis, MN 55415 1-800-321-BURN (2876) 612-347-2915 612-347-6036 fax
	St. Paul	Ramsey Burn Center St. Paul–Ramsey Medical Center 640 Jackson Street St. Paul, MN 55101 612-221-3351 612-292-4040 fax
Mississippi	Greenville	Mississippi Firefighters Memorial Burn Center 1400 East Union Avenue Greenville, MS 38703 601-334-2514 601-334-2425 fax

Missouri	Columbia	University of Missouri–Columbia Hospital and Clinics One Hospital Drive Columbia, MO 65212 314-882-7994 314-884-4611 fax
	Kansas City	Children's Mercy Hospital 2401 Gilham Road Kansas City, MO 64108 816-234-3520 816-234-3821 fax
	St. Louis	Barnes Hospital Burn Center One Barnes Hospital Plaza St. Louis, MO 63110 314-362-4060
		St. John's Mercy Medical Center 615 South New Ballas Road St. Louis, MO 63141 314-569-6055 314-569-6910 fax
	Springfield	St. John's Regional Burn Unit 1235 East Cherokee Street Springfield, MO 65804-2263 417-885-2876 417-888-7880 fax
Montana	Billings	St. Vincent Hospital and Health Center Box 35200 Billings, MT 59107-5200 406-657-7067 406-657-7580 fax
Nebraska	Lincoln	St. Elizabeth Community Health Center Burn Center 555 South 70th Street Lincoln, NE 68510 402-486-7680 402-467-5457 fax

Nevada	Las Vegas	University Medical Center of Southern Nevada 1800 West Charleston Boulevard Las Vegas, NV 89102 702-383-2268
New Jersey	Hackensack	Hackensack Medical Center 30 Prospect Avenue Hackensack, NJ 07601 201-996-2000 201-342-9324 fax
	Livingston	Saint Barnabas Medical Center Old Short Hills Road Livingston, NJ 07039 201-533-5920 201-533-8089 fax
New Mexico	Albuquerque	University of New Mexico Regional Burn Center 2211 Lomas Boulevard, NE Albuquerque, NM 87106 505-843-2715 505-272-6493 fax
New York	Buffalo	Erie County Medical Center Burn Treatment Center 462 Grider Street Buffalo, NY 14215 716-898-5231 800-729-LIFE (Transfers) 716-898-5029 fax
	East Meadow	Burn Center Nassau County Medical Center 2201 Hempstead Turnpike East Meadow, NY 11554 516-742-3207 516-742-0257 fax
	Elmira	St. Joseph's Hospital Burn Unit 555 East Market Street Elmira, NY 14902 607-733-6541 607-737-7837 fax

(*continued*)

New York (*cont'd*)

	New York (Bronx)	Jacobi Hospital Burn Center Pelham Parkway S. and Eastchester Road Bronx, NY 10461 718-918-6606 718-918-5567 fax
	New York (Manhattan)	New York Hospital Burn Center 525 East 68th Street New York, NY 10021 212-746-5317 212-746-8991 fax
	Rochester	Strong Memorial Hospital 601 Elmwood Avenue Rochester, NY 14642 716-275-5471 716-271-5739 fax
	Stony Brook	Burn Center–University Hospital State University of New York at Stony Brook Stony Brook, NY 11794 516-444-2270
	Syracuse	Burn Unit SUNY Health Science Center 750 East Adams Street Syracuse, NY 13210 315-464-6083 315-464-6238 fax
	Valhalla	Westchester Burn Center Westchester County Medical Center Grasslands Road Valhalla, NY 10595 914-285-8677 914-285-7806 fax
	West Islip	Good Samaritan Hospital 800 Montauk Highway West Islip, NY 11795 516-661-3000 516-669-3818

North Carolina	Chapel Hill	North Carolina Jaycee Burn Center The Hospitals at the University of North Carolina Chapel Hill, NC 27514 919-966-3571 919-966-5732 fax
	Durham	Duke University Hospital Box 3708 Durham, NC 27710 919-681-2404 919-681-8985 fax
	Winston-Salem	North Carolina Baptist Hospital Burn Unit Medical Center Boulevard Winston-Salem, NC 27157 919-716-7766 919-716-6300
North Dakota	Fargo	St. Luke's Hospitals–Meritcare 720 Fourth Street, South Fargo, ND 58122 701-234-5721 701-234-5197 fax
Ohio	Akron	Regional Burn Center Children's Hospital Medical Center of Akron 281 Locust Street Akron, OH 44308 216-379-8224 216-379-8152 fax
	Cincinnati	Shriners Burns Institute 3229 Burnet Avenue Cincinnati, OH 45229-3095 513-872-6000 513-872-6999 fax
		University of Cincinnati Hospital 234 Goodman Street Cincinnati, OH 45219 513-558-8199 513-558-3474 fax

(*continued*)

Ohio (*cont'd*)

	Cleveland	MetroHealth Medical Center Burn Unit 2500 MetroHealth Drive Cleveland, OH 44109 216-459-5643 216-459-5616 fax
	Columbus	Burn Unit Children's Hospital 700 Children's Drive Columbus, OH 43205 614-461-2560 614-461-2633 fax
		Ohio State University Hospitals 410 West Tenth Avenue Columbus, OH 43210-1228 614-293-8744
	Dayton	Miami Valley Hospital Regional Adult Burn Unit One Wyoming Street Dayton, OH 45409-2722 513-220-2126 513-220-2450 fax
	Toledo	Northwest Ohio Regional Burn Care and Reconstructive Center St. Vincent Medical Center 2213 Cherry Street Toledo, OH 43608-2691 419-321-4734 419-321-3286 fax
Oklahoma	Oklahoma City	Baptist Burn Center 3300 Northwest Expressway Oklahoma City, OK 73112 405-949-3345 405-949-3662 fax
		Children's Hospital of Oklahoma Burn Services 940 NE 13th Street Oklahoma City, OK 73104 405-271-4733 405-271-3017

	Tulsa	Alexander Burn Center Hillcrest Medical Center 1120 South Utica Tulsa, OK 74104 918-579-4590 918-579-2223 fax
Oregon	Portland	Oregon Burn Center Emanuel Hospital 2801 North Gantenbein Avenue Portland, OR 97227 503-280-4232
Pennsylvania	Allentown	Burn Center–Lehigh Valley Hospital Center Cedar Crest and I-78 P.O. Box 689 Allentown, PA 18105-1556 215-402-8735 215-402-8734 215-402-1674 fax
	Erie	Hamot Medical Center 201 State Street Erie, PA 16550-0001 814-877-6130 814-877-6188 fax
	Philadelphia	Saint Agnes Medical Center 1900 South Broad Street Philadelphia, PA 19145 215-339-4339 215-339-0482 fax
		St. Christopher's Hospital for Children Pediatric Burn Center Erie Avenue at Front Street Philadelphia, PA 19134-1095 215-427-5000 215-427-5555 fax

(*continued*)

Pennsylvania (*cont'd*)		
	Pittsburgh	Mercy Hospital of Pittsburgh 1400 Locust Street Pittsburgh, PA 15219 412-232-8225 412-232-8134 fax
		The Western Pennsylvania Hospital Burn-Trauma Center 4800 Friendship Avenue Pittsburgh, PA 15224 412-578-5273 412-578-4934 fax
	Upland	The Nathan Speare Regional Burn Treatment Center Crozer-Chester Medical Center One Medical Center Boulevard Upland, PA 19013-3995 215-447-2800 215-872-4015 fax
South Carolina	Charleston	Medical University of South Carolina Burn Center 171 Ashley Avenue Charleston, SC 29425 803-792-3681 803-792-3159 fax
		Pediatric Burn Center The Children's Hospital Medical University Medical Center 171 Ashley Avenue Charleston, SC 29425 803-792-2123 803-792-3858 fax
South Dakota	Sioux Falls	McKennan Hospital Burn Unit 800 East 21st Street Sioux Falls, SD 57101 605-333-8425 605-339-7543 fax

Tennessee	Chattanooga	Erlanger Medical Center Burn Unit 975 East Third Street Chattanooga, TN 37406 615-778-7881 615-778-7708 fax
	Memphis	Regional Burn Center at Memphis 877 Jefferson Avenue Memphis, TN 38103 901-575-8090 901-575-7816 fax
	Nashville	Burn Center Vanderbilt University Hospital S-4400 RW Medical Center North Nashville, TN 37232-2165 615-322-4590 615-343-6873 fax
Texas	Dallas	Parkland Memorial Hospital 5301 Harry Hines Boulevard P.O. Box 45188 Dallas, TX 75235 214-590-7650 214-590-5402 fax
	El Paso	Sun Towers Hospital 1801 North Oregon Street El Paso, TX 79902 915-521-1780 915-533-2083
	Galveston	Shriners Burns Institute 815 Market Street Galveston, TX 77550 409-770-6600 409-770-6749 fax
		Blocker Burn Intensive Care Unit University of Texas Medical Branch Eighth and Mechanic Streets Galveston, TX 77550 409-761-2023 409-761-5112 fax

(*continued*)

Texas (*cont'd*)		
	Houston	Hermann Hospital 6411 Fannin Street Houston, TX 77030-1501 713-797-4350 713-792-4294 fax
	Lubbock	Timothy J. Harnar Burn Center University Medical Center P.O. Box 5980 602 Indiana Avenue Lubbock, TX 79417 806-743-3406 800-345-9911 806-743-1946 fax
	San Antonio	St. Luke's Lutheran Hospital Burn Unit P.O. Box 29100 7930 Floyd Curl Drive San Antonio, TX 78229-0100 210-517-7000 210-692-3337 fax
		US Army Institute of Surgical Research Fort Sam Houston, TX 78234-5012 512-222-BURN (2876) 512-271-0830 fax
Utah	Salt Lake City	Intermountain Burn Center University of Utah Medical Center 50 North Medical Drive Salt Lake City, UT 84132 801-581-2700 801-585-2103 fax
Vermont	Burlington	Medical Center Hospital of Vermont Burn Program Colchester Avenue Burlington, VT 05404 802-656-2434 802-656-5342 fax

Virginia	Charlottesville	DeCamp Burn Center University of Virginia Health Sciences Center Lee Street Charlottesville, VA 22908 804-924-BURN (2876) 804-924-8299 fax
	Norfolk	Sentara Norfolk General Hospital Burn Center 600 Gresham Drive Norfolk, VA 23507 804-628-3117 804-628-3437 fax
	Richmond	Medical College of Virginia/Virginia Commonwealth University Burn Unit Box 7, MCV Station Richmond, VA 23298 804-786-9240 804-371-7710 fax
Washington	Bellingham	St. Joseph's Hospital 2901 Squalicum Parkway Bellingham, WA 98225 206-734-5400 x3501
	Seattle	University of Washington Burn Center at Harborview Medical Center 325 Ninth Avenue, ZA-16 Seattle, WA 98104 206-284-BURN (2876) 206-223-3656 fax
	Spokane	Sacred Heart Medical Center West 101 8th Avenue TAF C9 Spokane, WA 99204 509-455-4644
	Tacoma	Firefighters Burn Center St. Joseph Hospital and Health Care Center 1718 South I Street Tacoma, WA 98405 206-591-6677

West Virginia	Huntington	Cabell Huntington Hospital–Burn Unit 1340 Hal Greer Boulevard Huntington, WV 25704 304-526-2390 304-526-2008 fax
Wisconsin	Madison	University of Wisconsin Hospital and Clinics 600 Highland Avenue Madison, WI 53792 608-263-1490 608-263-7652 fax
	Milwaukee	St. Mary's Regional Burn Center 2323 North Lake Drive Milwaukee, WI 53211 414-291-1000 414-291-1495 fax
		CANADA
Alberta	Calgary	Alberta Children's Hospital 1820 Richmond Road, SW Calgary, Alberta, T2T 5C7 403-229-7890 403-229-7221 fax
		Burn Treatment Centre Foothills Hospital 1403 29 Street, NW Calgary, Alberta T2N 2T9 403-670-1110
	Edmonton	Firefighters Burn Treatment Unit University of Alberta Hospitals 4C2 WMHSC 8440-112th Street Edmonton, Alberta T6G 2B7 403-492-6149 403-492-4923 fax

British Columbia	Vancouver	Burn Unit Vancouver General Hospital 855 West 12th Avenue Vancouver, British Columbia V5Z 1M9 604-875-4030 604-875-5614 fax
	Victoria	Royal Jubilee Hospital Burn Unit 1900 Fort Street Victoria, British Columbia V8R 1J8 604-595-9271
Manitoba	Winnipeg	Burn Unit–CK3 Winnipeg Children's Hospital 840 Sherbrook Street Winnipeg, Manitoba R3A 1S1 204-787-4785 204-787-4807 fax
		Health Sciences Center Ward GH5 820 Sherbrook Street Winnipeg, Manitoba R3A 1R9 204-787-3775 204-787-5002 fax
New Brunswick	Moncton	The Moncton Hospital Burn Unit, 6400 Unit 135 MacBeath Avenue Moncton, New Brunswick E1C 6Z8 506-857-5527
	St. John	Burn and Plastic Surgery Unit St. John Regional Hospital St. John, New Brunswick E2L 4L2 506-648-6176

Nova Scotia	Halifax	Burn Unit/7 North Victoria General Hospital 1278 Tower Road Halifax, Nova Scotia B3H 1Y5 902-428-2525 902-428-2558 fax
		Izaak Walton Killiam Children's Hospital P.O. Box 3070 Halifax, Nova Scotia B3J 3G9 902-428-8350 902-428-8826 fax
Ontario	Hamilton	Firefighter's Burn Trauma Unit Hamilton General Hospital 237 Barton Street, East Hamilton, Ontario L8L 2X2 416-527-0271 ext. 6350 416-527-1941 fax
	Kingston	Shriner Burn Unit Hotel Dieu Hospital Kingston, Ontario K7L 5G2 613-544-3310 ext. 2461 613-544-9897 fax
	London	Thompson Burn Unit Victoria Hospital 375 South Street London, Ontario N6A 4G5 519-685-8500 ext. 5735
	Ottawa	Children's Hospital of Eastern Ontario 401 Smyth Road Ottawa, Ontario K1H 8L1 613-737-7600 613-738-4840 fax
	Scarborough	Scarborough General Hospital Scarborough, Ontario M1P 2V5 416-438-2911 416-438-9318 fax

	Toronto	The Burn Unit - 8th Floor Atrium The Hospital for Sick Children 555 University Avenue Toronto, Ontario M5G 1X8 416-813-6932 416-598-7505 fax
		Wellesley Burn Centre Wellesley Hospital 160 Wellesley Street, E Toronto, Ontario M4Y 1J3 416-926-7021 416-926-7603 fax
	Windsor	Essex County Regional Burn Unit Metropolitan General Hospital 1995 Lens Avenue Windsor, Ontario N8W 1L9 519-254-1661 x2334 519-254-0883 fax
Quebec	Montreal	Burn Unit–Montreal Children's Hospital 2300 Tupper Street Montreal, Quebec H3H 1P3 514-934-4400 514-934-4477 fax
		Montreal General Hospital 1650 Cedar Avenue Montreal, Quebec H3G 1A4 514-937-6011 514-934-8203
Saskatchewan	Regina	South Saskatchewan Fire Fighters' Burn Unit Regina General Hospital 1440 14th Avenue Regina, Saskatchewan S4P 0W5 306-359-4648 306-359-4256 306-359-4723 fax

(*continued*)

Saskatchewan (*cont'd*)		
	Saskatoon	Burn Unit Royal University Hospital Saskatoon, Saskatchewan S7N 0X0 306-966-1891 306-966-1660 fax

Glossary

Adaptive equipment Modifications of utensils to make their use easier.

ADL (activities of daily living) Activities that enable a person to meet everyday needs; includes feeding, dressing, and bathing.

Albumin A protein often given intravenously in resuscitation.

Ambulation Walking.

Analgesia Decreased sensation induced by administration of an analgesic.

Anesthesia Absence of sensation induced by administration of an anesthetic.

General A sleep-like state.

Spinal An anesthetic agent injected in the back to put the lower body to sleep.

Anesthesiologist/anesthetist A specialist in anesthesia.

Arterial line (A-line) A hollow tube placed in an artery to measure blood pressure.

Automatic intravenous infusion pump A device for pumping fluids through intravenous lines.

Bandage

Ace A brand of elastic bandage.

Kerlix A brand of bandage.

Kling A brand of bandage.

Beds

Air bed See "Air-fluidized bed."

Air-fluidized bed Bed containing myriads of small air-blown beads, on which the patient floats to reduce pressure on the back.

Clinitron Brand of air-fluidized bed.

Flexicare Brand of special low-pressure bed with air-insufflated rubber mattresses under the patient.

Kinair Brand of air-fluidized bed.

Bronchoscopy A procedure in which the physician looks down the airway and lungs with a special magnified, lighted tube; used in the diagnosis of smoke inhalation and in the treatment of pneumonia.

Burn

Chemical A burn induced by a chemical agent.

Contact A burn caused by direct contact with a hot object.

Electrical An injury caused by electricity.

First degree A superficial burn injuring only the epidermis.

Flame A burn caused by burning objects, i.e., flame.

Flash A burn caused by a sudden flash of heat or fire but without anything catching fire.

Scald A burn caused by hot liquid.

Second degree A partial-thickness burn injuring part of the dermis as well as the epidermis.

Third degree A burn destroying all of the epidermis and all of the dermis.

Capillaries Small vessels that exchange blood between arteries and veins.

Capsulectomy Surgical removal of the joint capsule to release ligaments around a joint.

Cardiologist A specialist in treating the heart.

Catheter A hollow tube introduced into an organ.

Bladder A tube inserted into the bladder usually to measure urine output accurately.

Foley A brand of bladder catheter.

Swan-Ganz A tube inserted through a vein into the heart to measure pressures.

Urinary Same as bladder catheter.

Compression garment An elastic garment made and worn to apply gentle pressure to healing burns to reduce scarring.

Consent form A form presented by staff to a patient or next of kin, which must be understood and signed before any procedure such as a surgical operation can be done on the patient.

Dangling Sitting on the edge of the bed or chair with legs in a dependent position; first step toward walking (process of placing leg down to regain normal circulation).

Debridement Removal or clearing of dead tissue, old creams, secretions, etc. from the burn wound.

Depigmentation Loss of skin color from burn damage to skin cells.

Dermis The second layer of skin, under the epidermis.

Dialysis Treatment on the artificial kidney, applied in case of kidney failure.

Disposition What happens to a patient at discharge, i.e., home, nursing home, etc.

Donor area A part of the body from which skin grafts are taken to cover the burn.

Dressings
- **Adaptic** Brand name for a nonadherent finely meshed gauze.
- **Burn** Very thick, coarse-mesh gauze.
- **Kerlix** Brand name for a two-way stretch gauze bandage.
- **Kling** Brand name for a one-way stretch gauze bandage.
- **Scarlet red** A dressing impregnated with the red antiseptic dye scarlet red.
- **Wet-to-dry** Dressings placed wet, allowed to dry, then removed.
- **Wet-to-wet** Dressing placed wet, kept wet, and changed wet.

Edema Swelling.

Electrocardiogram (EKG) Electrical tracing of heart function.

Endotracheal (ET) tube Breathing tube placed into the windpipe through the nose or mouth.

Epidermis The top layer of the skin.

Epithelialization Natural division and multiplication of skin cells to cover a wound.

Eschar Dead skin and underlying tissue.

Escharotomy An incision in the burn through skin to the underlying fat.

Excision Surgical removal of the eschar.
- **Fascial** The eschar is removed to a deep, even level.
- **Tangential** The eschar is sliced away until all the dead tissue is removed.

Expander A balloon placed under healthy skin to stretch it for use as donor area.

Flap Portion of healthy tissue used to cover a damaged area.
- **Distant** A flap moved to an area not adjacent to the donor site.
- **Free** A flap whose blood supply is other than the donor site.

Local A flap moved to an area adjacent to the donor site.

Gait training Training to achieve a normal pattern of walking.

Gases Blood tests used to measure adequacy of respiration.

Gastrointestinal tract Body system that provides digestion of food.

Goniometer Device used to measure angles of motion of joints.

Graft Portion of tissue placed to cover a damaged area at some distance.
Composite A graft containing more than one type of tissue.
Full thickness The whole skin is used; the resulting defect is surgically closed.
Split thickness Partial-thickness skin is used; the resulting defect heals by itself.

Heat shield A heat-radiating device used to keep people warm.

Heterotopic ossification Buildup of bone across a joint where bone is not usually present.

Hydrotherapy Treatment by water (bath, spa, spray, arm or foot tank, etc.).

Inhalation Breathing in smoke or products of smoke.

Inhalation injury Airway injury by inhalation.

Intensive care unit (ICU) The unit of the hospital where critically ill patients are treated.

Intravenous (IV) Injection, fluid, or medication given into a vein.
Central An IV given into a large vein usually in the neck or groin.
Peripheral An IV given into a small vein in the arm or foot.

Intubate To place a plastic tube into the windpipe to help breathing.

Isokinetic exercise Exercise for strengthening in which muscle works against a set speed.

Lines
Intraarterial See "Arterial line."
Intravenous Sterile tube in a vein (see IV).

Lumbar puncture A diagnostic test; a needle is inserted into the backbone to draw out spinal fluid.

Mesh Donor skin with holes punched in it and expanded.

Monitor A machine that shows vital functions electrically and sounds an alarm if they are abnormal.

Mouth retractor Devices to increase opening width of mouth.

MRI (magnetic resonance imaging) A technique creating images using magnetic fields.

Muscle atrophy Loss of muscle bulk due to immobility.

Myositis ossificans Buildup of bone in a muscle.

Nasopharyngoscopy Inspection of the nose and throat with a flexible electric light.

Nephrologist A specialist in the treatment of the kidneys.

Neurologist A nerve specialist.

Operating room A special area in the hospital for surgical operations.

Oral commissures The sides of the mouth where the lips come together.

Orthostatic hypotension Rapid drop in blood pressure when standing up following bed rest.

Osteoporosis Loss of bone density.

Oxygen Normal component of air, often given to patients in high concentrations.

Passive ROM Exercise in which a joint is moved through the range of motion by another person.

Pediatrician A specialist in the care of children.

Physical and occupational therapy Medical specialties that provide rehabilitation through the use of physical modalities, exercise, and splinting.

Pigmentation Skin color, sometimes lost following burns.

Plasma The liquid part of blood.

Platelets Tiny blood cells, smaller than red cells, which help to stop bleeding.

Pressure sores Breakdown of skin areas due to constant pressure.

Procedure Anything that a doctor or nurse does to a patient which breaks the skin: e.g., an operation, the insertion of a tube, the starting of an IV.

Prognosis Outlook.

Psychiatrist A specialist in the treatment of mental disturbances who is licensed to prescribe medications.

Psychologist A specialist in the treatment of mental disturbances.

Pulmonary Having to do with the lungs.

Pulse oximeter The part of the monitor which measures oxygen levels in the blood.

Range of motion (ROM) Distance through which a joint can move.

Active assisted ROM Exercise in which the patient moves the joint through the range of motion with the help of another person.

Active ROM Exercise in which the patient moves the joint through the range of motion without help.

Contracture Limitation of motion caused by skin, muscle, and/or joint tightness.

Strength Measurement of how strongly a muscle can move.

Recipient area The area of skin destroyed by burn which will receive the donor skin during grafting.

Red cells The cellular, or solid, part of the blood—suspended in plasma.

Rehabilitation The process by which an injured person regains function for return to normal daily activity.

Renal Having to do with the kidneys.

Resistive exercise Exercise for strengthening in which a muscle works against a weight.

Respirator A breathing machine.

Respiratory insufficiency Inadequate function of the lungs; usually requires a respirator for treatment.

Resting skin tension lines (RSTL) The natural contours of the face and body.

Scan Creation of an image of an internal organ by x-ray, magnetic rays, or other techniques.

Cat scan A precise form of x-ray; gives a clearer image than ordinary x-rays.

Scar

Contracture A scar formed when tissue shortens, causing deformity and limitation of motion.

Hypertrophic Scar formation abnormally thickened and hard.

Keloid Like a hypertrophic scar but even thicker and harder, and extending beyond the original site of the scar.

Pathological Any scar that results in dysfunction or deformity.

Sepsis Infection.

Shock Low blood pressure and poor circulation.

Skin graft

- Allograft A graft from a different individual to a patient.
- Artificial skin Skin substitute that contains partly or wholly synthetic or animal material.
- Cultured skin Skin grown in the test tube from a small piece of a patient's own uninjured skin.
- Donor site The part of the body where the skin graft was taken from.
- Heterograft Same as Xenograft.
- Homograft Same as Allograft.
- Recipient site The area of burn where the skin graft is placed.
- Xenograft A graft from a different species; e.g., pigskin applied to a person.

Splint A static or dynamic device used to position a body area.

Staples Small metal clips sometimes used to hold grafts in place.

Step-down An area of the burn unit where less acute care is given.

Suction A device in intensive care rooms to apply negative pressure: clear secretions from lungs, stomach contents, etc.

Sutures (Also stitches) Dissolving or permanent threads used to secure grafts, to close donor sites, and for other repairs.

Tissue expansion A technique for increasing the amount of local tissue available for flaps.

Tracheostomy An opening in the windpipe, made by surgeons to make the patient's breathing more comfortable.

Transfer The process of moving a person from one place to another when person is not able to walk.

Transparent mask/splint A device used for scar pressure which is clear and see-through.

Tubbing Immersion in a large water bath for the purpose of cleaning the burn.

Tubes

- Chest Placed in the chest cavity to relieve an air leak or bleeding or to drain fluid.
- Endotracheal Placed in the windpipe to help with breathing.
- Jejunostomy Placed in the bowel for feeding.

Nasogastric Placed in the stomach through the nose or mouth to keep the stomach empty or for feeding.

Tracheostomy Placed in the windpipe (see "Tracheostomy").

Unna boot A supportive dressing for the foot and leg.

Ventilator See "Respirator."

Vital capacity The amount of oxygen that can be exchanged in a lung during breathing.

W-plasty A type of local skin flap.

Wall sockets Source of the oxygen and air delivered to the patient in the hospital as well as a source of suction for clearing body fluids.

Web spacers Devices used to increase or maintain area in between fingers.

Z-plasty A type of local skin flap.

Index